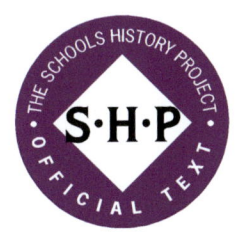

OCR SHP GCSE

THE PEOPLE'S HEALTH

c.1250 TO PRESENT

JAMIE BYROM
MICHAEL RILEY

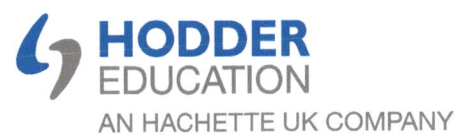

The Schools History Project

Set up in 1972 to bring new life to history for school students, the Schools History Project has been based at Leeds Trinity University since 1978. SHP continues to play an innovatory role in history education based on its six principles:

- Making history meaningful for young people
- Engaging in historical enquiry
- Developing broad and deep knowledge
- Studying the historic environment
- Promoting diversity and inclusion
- Supporting rigorous and enjoyable learning

These principles are embedded in the resources which SHP produces in partnership with Hodder Education to support history at Key Stage 3, GCSE (SHP OCR B) and A level. The Schools History Project contributes to national debate about school history. It strives to challenge, support and inspire teachers through its published resources, conferences and website: http://www.schoolshistoryproject.co.uk

This resource is endorsed by OCR for use with specification OCR Level 1/2 GCSE (9–1) in History B (Schools History Project) (J411). In order to gain OCR endorsement, this resource has undergone an independent quality check. Any references to assessment and/or assessment preparation are the publisher's interpretation of the specification requirements and are not endorsed by OCR. OCR recommends that a range of teaching and learning resources are used in preparing learners for assessment. OCR has not paid for the production of this resource, nor does OCR receive any royalties from its sale. For more information about the endorsement process, please visit the OCR website, www.ocr.org.uk.

The publishers thank OCR for permission to use specimen exam questions on pages 104–105 from OCR's GCSE (9–1) History B (Schools History Project) © OCR 2016. OCR have neither seen nor commented upon any model answers or exam guidance related to these questions.

Every effort has been made to trace all copyright holders, but if any have been inadvertently overlooked, the Publishers will be pleased to make the necessary arrangements at the first opportunity.

Although every effort has been made to ensure that website addresses are correct at time of going to press, Hodder Education cannot be held responsible for the content of any website mentioned in this book. It is sometimes possible to find a relocated web page by typing in the address of the home page for a website in the URL window of your browser.

Orders: please contact Hachette UK Distribution, Hely Hutchinson Centre, Milton Road, Didcot, Oxfordshire, OX11 7HH. Telephone: +44 (0)1235 827827. Email education@hachette.co.uk Lines are open from 9 a.m. to 5 p.m., Monday to Friday. You can also order through our website: www.hoddereducation.co.uk

ISBN: 978 1 4718 6008 9

© Jamie Byrom, Michael Riley 2016

First published in 2016 by
Hodder Education,
An Hachette UK Company
Carmelite House
50 Victoria Embankment
London EC4Y 0DZ

www.hoddereducation.co.uk

The authorised representative in the EEA is Hachette Ireland, 8 Castlecourt Centre, Dublin 15, D15 XTP3, Ireland (email: info@hbgi.ie)

Impression number   10 9 8 7 6
Year   2023

All rights reserved. Apart from any use permitted under UK copyright law, no part of this publication may be reproduced or transmitted in any form or by any means, electronic or mechanical, including photocopying and recording, or held within any information storage and retrieval system, without permission in writing from the publisher or under licence from the Copyright Licensing Agency Limited. Further details of such licences (for reprographic reproduction) may be obtained from the Copyright Licensing Agency Limited, www.cla.co.uk

Cover photo: © Photo Researchers/Mary Evans Picture Library

Typeset by White-Thomson Publishing Ltd

Printed and bound by CPI Group (UK) Ltd, Croydon, CR0 4YY

A catalogue record for this title is available from the British Library.

CONTENTS

	Introduction	2
	Making the most of this book	
1	**Matters of life and death**	8
	Did anyone really care about health in medieval England?	
	Closer look 1 – Exeter's medieval water supplies	
2	**The people's health, 1500–1750**	30
	More of the same?	
	Closer look 2 – The 1636 plague in Newcastle	
3	**Revolution!**	54
	Why were there such huge changes in the people's health, 1750–1900?	
	Closer look 3 – Joseph Bazalgette and the revolution in London's sewers	
4	**Better than ever?**	76
	Do the changes in public health since 1900 tell a simple story of progress?	
	Closer look 4 – Health: a global perspective	
	Preparing for the examination	98
	Glossary	106
	Index	108
	Acknowledgements	111

INTRODUCTION

Making the most of this book

 Where this book fits into your GCSE history course

The course
The GCSE history course you are following is made up of five different studies. These are shown in the table below. For each type of study you will follow one option. We have highlighted the option that this particular book helps you with.

OCR SHP GCSE B

Paper 1 1 ¾ hours	**British thematic study** • The People's Health • Crime and Punishment • Migrants to Britain	**20%**
	British depth study • The Norman Conquest • The Elizabethans • Britain in Peace and War	**20%**
Paper 2 1 hour	**History around us** • Any site that meets the given criteria.	**20%**
Paper 3 1 ¾ hours	**World period study** • Viking Expansion • The Mughal Empire • The Making of America	**20%**
	World depth study • The First Crusade • Aztecs and the Spanish Conquest • Living under Nazi Rule	**20%**

The British thematic study
The British thematic study takes just one theme in British history and traces the way it has developed from about 1250 to the present day. The point of this type of study is to remind you of the characteristic features of life in Britain across all those centuries and to strengthen your understanding of how and why things change or, perhaps, stay the same.

Introduction

As the table shows, you will be examined on your knowledge and understanding of the British thematic study as part of Paper 1. You can find out more about that on pages 104–105 at the back of the book.

The chart below shows exactly what the examination specification requires for this thematic study.

The People's Health, c.1250 to present

The specification divides this thematic study into four periods:

Periods	Learners should study the following content:
Medieval Britain, c.1250–c.1500	• The characteristic features of medieval Britain: an overview • Living conditions: housing, food, clean water and waste • Responses to the Black Death: beliefs and actions • Approaches to public health in late-medieval towns and monasteries
Early Modern Britain, c.1500–c.1750	• Cultural, social and economic change including the growth of towns: an overview • Changing living conditions: housing, food, clean water and waste • Responses to outbreaks of plague including national plague orders and local reactions • The impact of local and national government on public health including measures to improve the urban environment and the government response to the gin craze, 1660–1751
Industrial Britain, c.1750–c.1900	• Industrialisation, the growth of major cities and political change: an overview • Urban living conditions in the early nineteenth century: housing, food, clean water and waste • Responses to cholera epidemics • Public health reform in the nineteenth century including the Public Health Acts and local initiatives
Britain since c.1900	• Economic, political, social and cultural change: an overview • Living conditions and lifestyles: housing, food, air quality and inactivity • Responses to Spanish Influenza and AIDS • Growing government involvement in public health including pollution controls, anti-smoking initiatives and the promotion of healthy lifestyles

Issues and factors

The bullets in each period tackle similar **issues**:

- An overview of life in the period. This will not tell you directly about changes in health care, but it helps to explain the issues that follow.
- Living conditions and how they affected health
- Epidemics and how people at the time responded to them
- How governments and others in authority attempted to improve public health.

The specification also says you should be able to explain how each of five **factors** has affected the people's health:

1. Beliefs, attitudes and values
2. Local and national government
3. Science and technology
4. Urbanisation
5. Wealth and poverty

The next two pages show how this book works.

How this book works

The rest of this book (from page 6 to page 97) is carefully arranged to match what the specification requires. It does this through the following features:

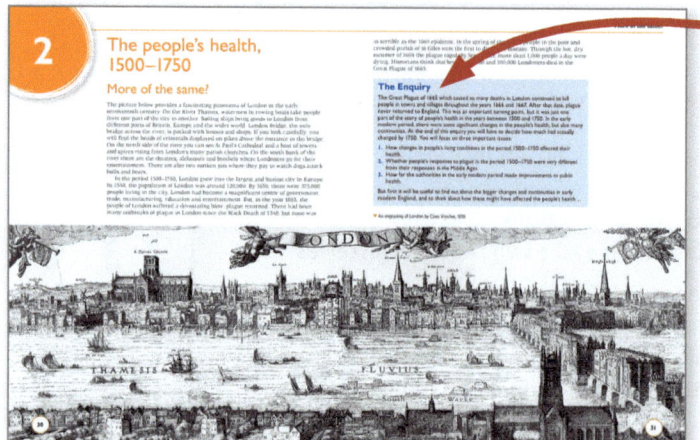

Enquiries

The book is largely taken up with four 'enquiries'. Each enquiry sets you a challenge in the form of an overarching question.

The first two pages of the enquiry set up the challenge and give you a clear sense of what you will need to do to work out your answer to the main question. You will find the instructions set out in 'The Enquiry' box, on a blue background, as in this example.

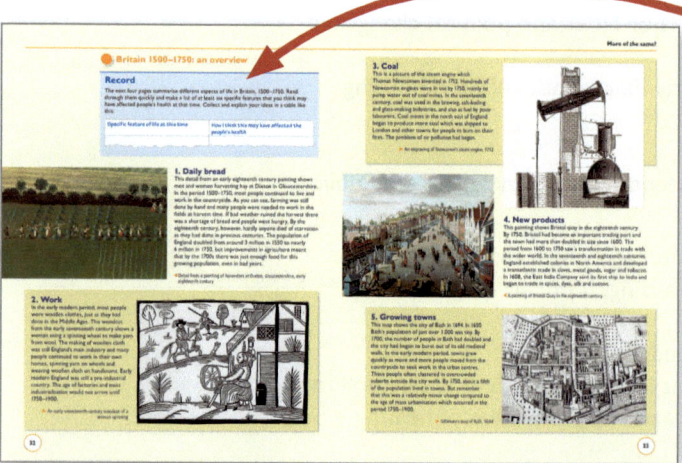

Record tasks

From that point, the enquiry is divided into four sections. These match the bullet points shown in the specification on page 3. You can tell when you are starting a new section as it will start with a large coloured heading like the one shown here. Throughout each section there are 'Record' tasks, where you will be asked to record ideas and information that will help you make up your mind about the overarching enquiry question later on. You can see an example of these 'Record' instructions here. They will always be in blue text with blue lines above and below them.

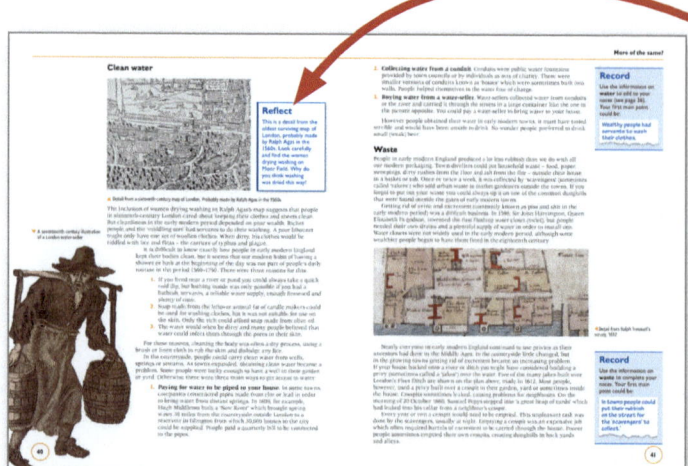

Reflect tasks

At regular intervals we will set a 'Reflect' task to prompt you to think carefully about what you are reading. They will look like the example shown here.

These Reflect tasks help you to check that what you are reading is making sense and to see how it connects with what you have already learned. You do not need to write down the ideas that you think of when you 'reflect', but the ideas you get may help you when you reach the next Record instruction.

Introduction

Review tasks

Each enquiry ends by asking you to review what you have been learning and use it to answer the overarching question in some way. Sometimes you simply answer that one question. Sometimes you will need to do two or three tasks that each tackle some aspect of the main question. The important point is that you should be able to use the ideas and evidence you have been building up through the enquiry to support your answer.

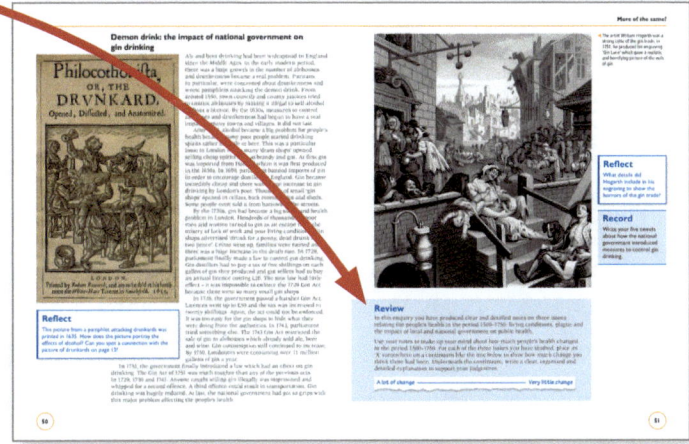

Closer looks

Between the enquiries you will find pages that provide a 'Closer look' at some aspect of the theme or period you are studying. These will often give you a chance to find out more about the issue you have just been studying in the previous enquiry, although they may sometimes look ahead to the next enquiry.

We may not include any tasks within these 'closer looks' but, as you read them, keep thinking of what they add to your knowledge and understanding. We think they add some intriguing insights.

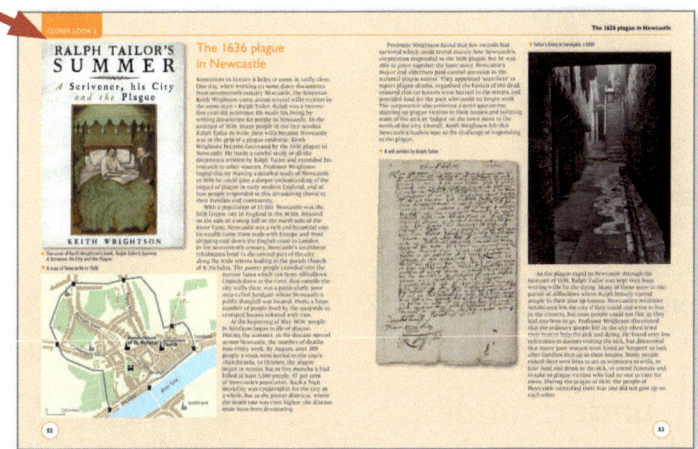

One very important final point

We have chosen enquiry questions that should help you get to the really important issues at the heart of each period you study, but you need to remember that the examiners will almost certainly ask you different questions when you take your GCSE. Don't simply rely on the notes you made to answer the enquiry question we gave you. We give you advice on how to tackle the examination and the different sorts of question you will face on pages 104–105.

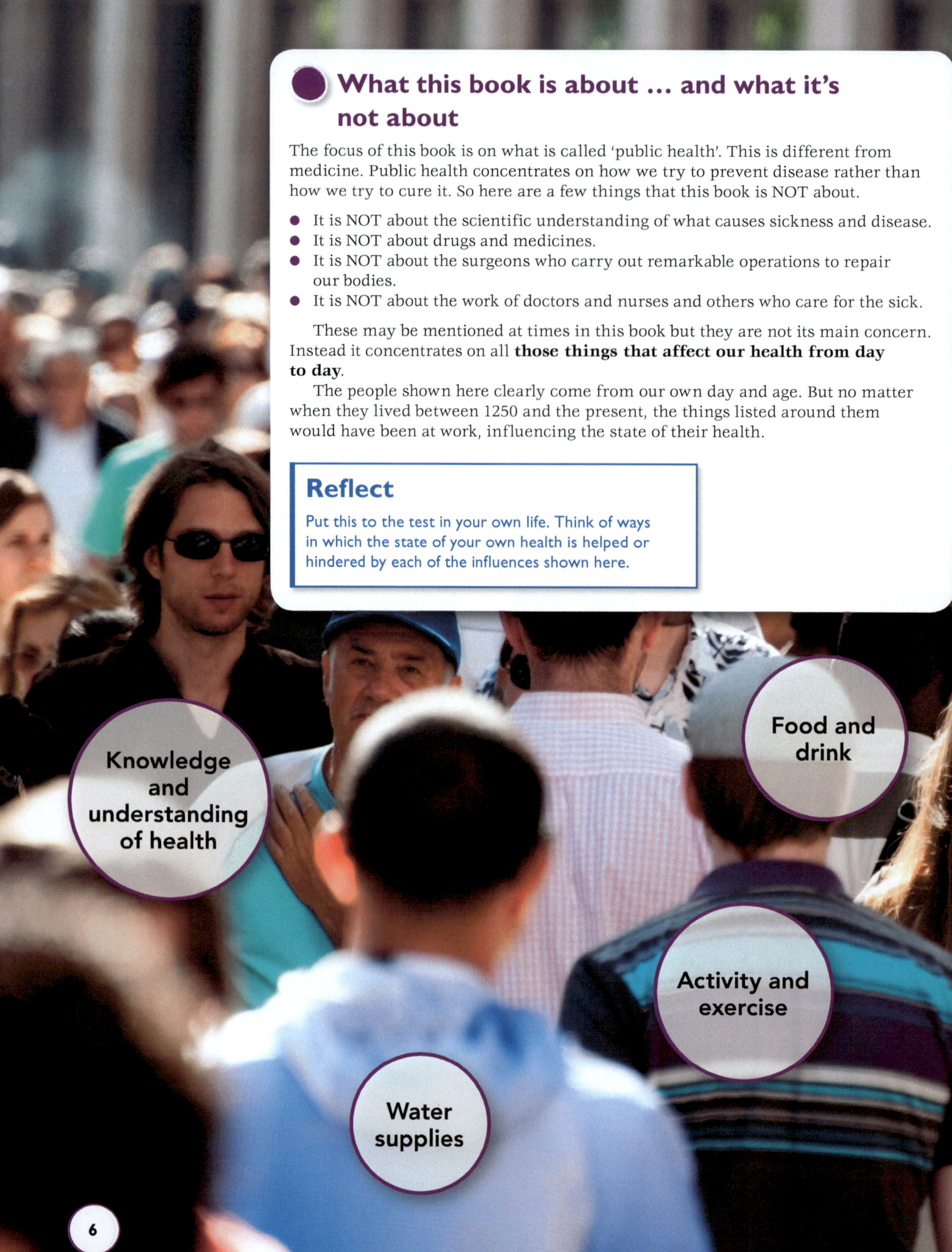

What this book is about … and what it's not about

The focus of this book is on what is called 'public health'. This is different from medicine. Public health concentrates on how we try to prevent disease rather than how we try to cure it. So here are a few things that this book is NOT about.

- It is NOT about the scientific understanding of what causes sickness and disease.
- It is NOT about drugs and medicines.
- It is NOT about the surgeons who carry out remarkable operations to repair our bodies.
- It is NOT about the work of doctors and nurses and others who care for the sick.

These may be mentioned at times in this book but they are not its main concern. Instead it concentrates on all **those things that affect our health from day to day**.

The people shown here clearly come from our own day and age. But no matter when they lived between 1250 and the present, the things listed around them would have been at work, influencing the state of their health.

Reflect

Put this to the test in your own life. Think of ways in which the state of your own health is helped or hindered by each of the influences shown here.

- Knowledge and understanding of health
- Food and drink
- Activity and exercise
- Water supplies

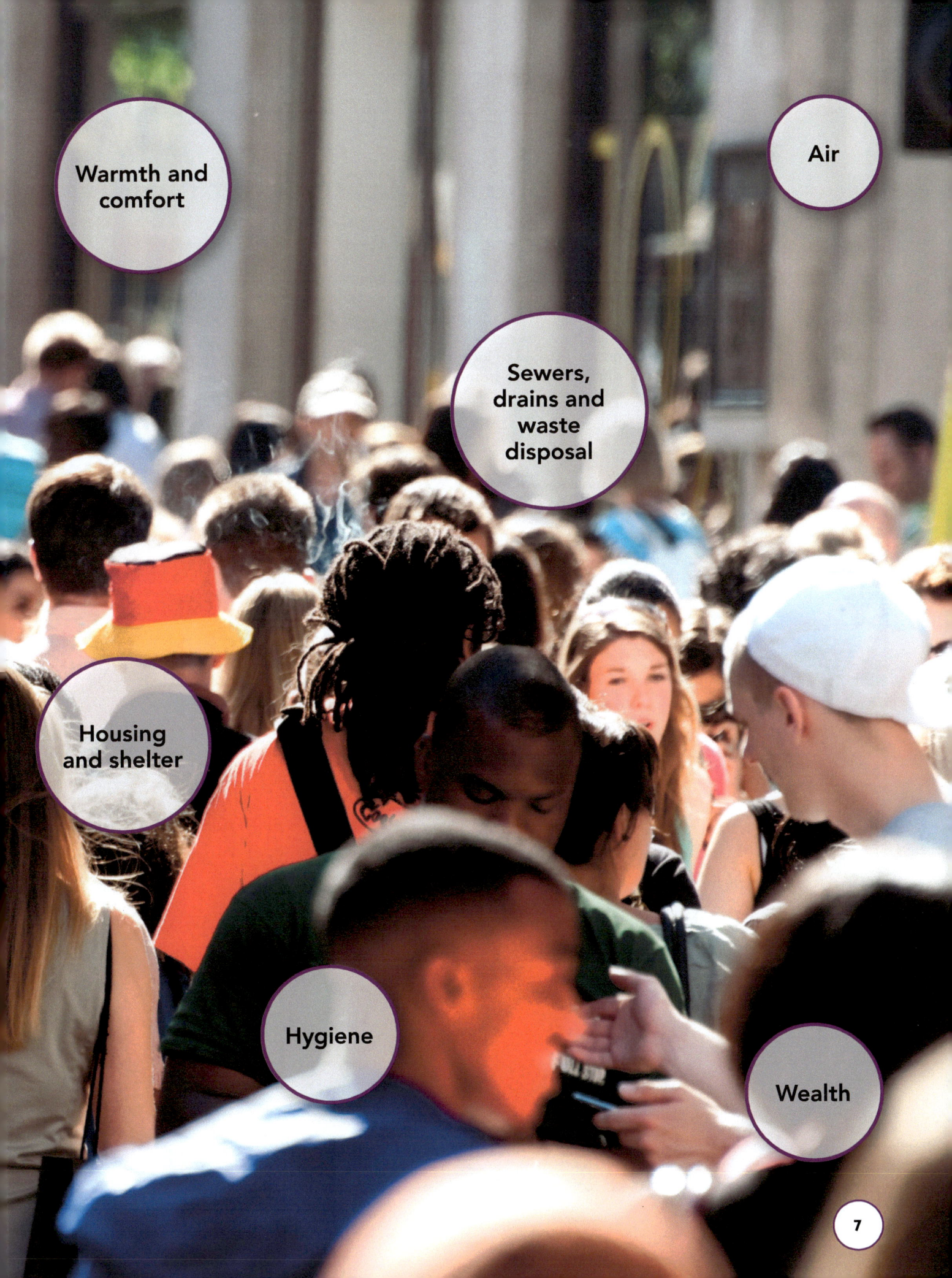

1 Matters of life and death

Did anyone really care about health in medieval England?

The image below appeared in 1976 in a magazine called *Look and Learn*. The magazine aimed to use interesting artwork to help young people learn about their world. This is an artist's impression of a London street scene in the fourteenth century.

If you were asked to look and learn from this picture, what impression would you get of whether anyone in medieval towns cared about their health?

▼ An illustration from *Look and Learn* magazine in 1976

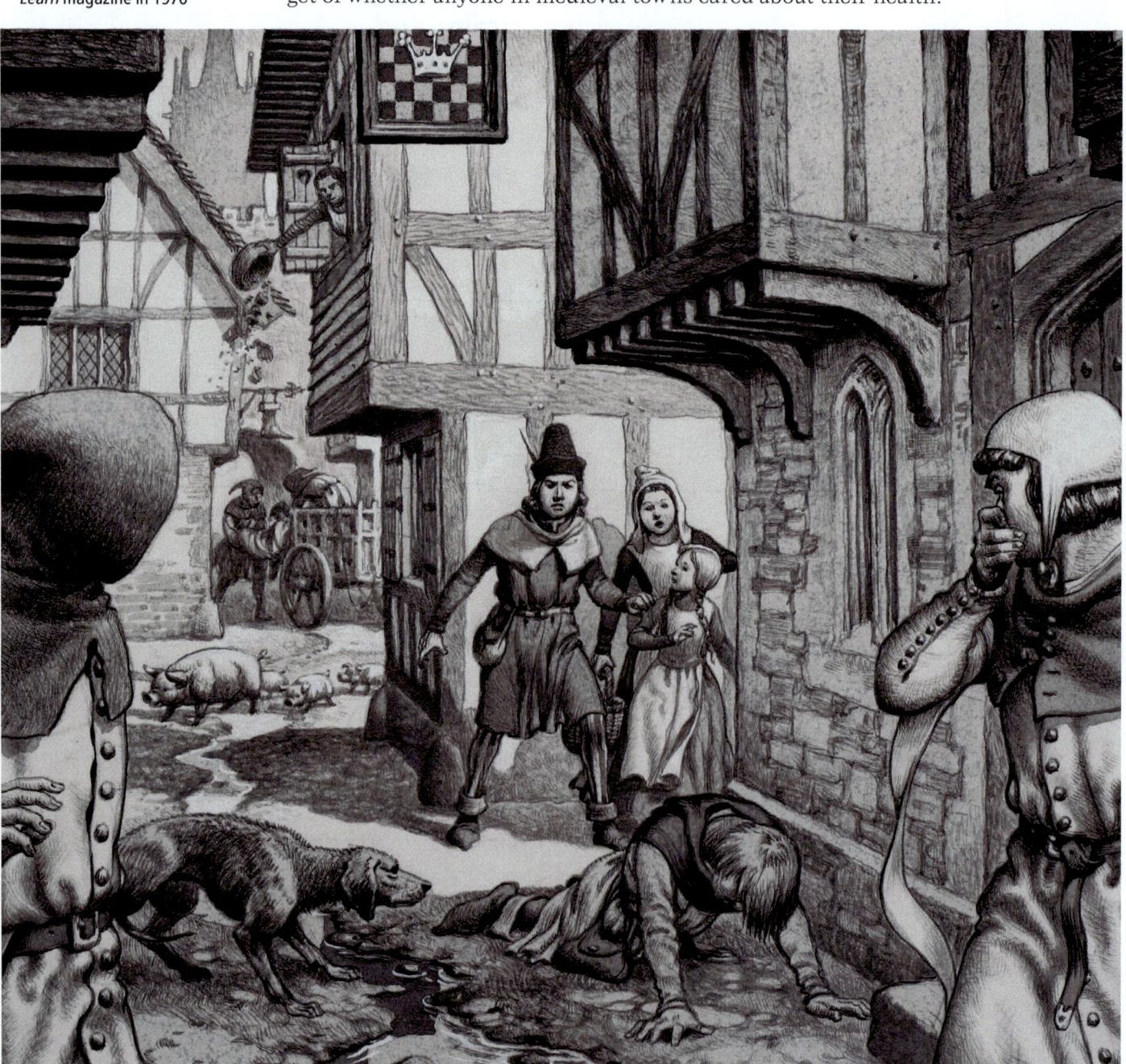

Did anyone really care about health in medieval England?

The Enquiry

The artist who created the image on page 8 has worked hard to create the impression that medieval towns were unhealthy places. A man suffering from deadly plague falls to his knees on the rough street. A dog sniffs at him suspiciously while fellow townspeople back away in alarm. These people show a perfectly natural fear of disease but apart from this, no one seems to care about the health of the city. A woman throws rubbish, or something worse, from an upstairs window and pigs roam freely through the city searching for food amidst the waste. The street itself has an open drain running through it. In the distance the body of another victim of plague, wrapped in a sheet, is being loaded onto a common cart by two hooded figures. The caption for the picture declared that *'London was such a filthy place at the time of the plague that nothing could be done to stop the disease'*.

It is certainly true that London in the Middle Ages was, by the standards of our own time, both dirty and full of dangers to health. But why was this? It is easy to assume that medieval people simply did not care about their health or that they were too stupid to take actions that seem obvious to us today. Your challenge in this enquiry is to decide whether medieval people made any serious effort to tackle the health hazards that faced cities, towns and villages in the period between 1250 and 1500. You will do this in four stages:

1. You will remind yourself about life in England in the Middle Ages.
2. You will learn about the conditions in which medieval people lived and consider whether or not they took care to avoid disease.
3. You will consider how people responded to the dreadful plague that first struck Britain in 1348. They knew it as the 'Great Pestilence' but it has since been called the Black Death.
4. Finally, you will find out exactly what those in authority, such as kings, church leaders and mayors, did to preserve the health of the people.

You will begin the first of these four stages on the next page. You will be reminding yourself how people lived in the Middle Ages and what they believed about their world. We call this wider knowledge the 'historical context'.

Fortunately we have a wonderful historical source to help us to get a sense of life in medieval Britain. It is the Luttrell Psalter, a collection of bible verses, prayers and other material that was made between 1320 and 1340 for a medieval knight called Sir Geoffrey Luttrell. Like all books of that time it was written and illustrated by hand.

On the right you can see a page from the psalter with its Bible verses in Latin surrounded by a delightful border of flowers and a curious fish with a human face. Beneath the writing, the monk has shown Sir Geoffrey on his splendid horse as his wife and sister-in-law hand him his lance and shield.

Every page of the psalter has a similar decoration of flowers, curious creatures and scenes from the world of Sir Geoffrey Luttrell and the people who lived on his lands in Lincolnshire. On the next four pages you will examine just ten of its many wonderful images to help you understand this wider context of medieval life.

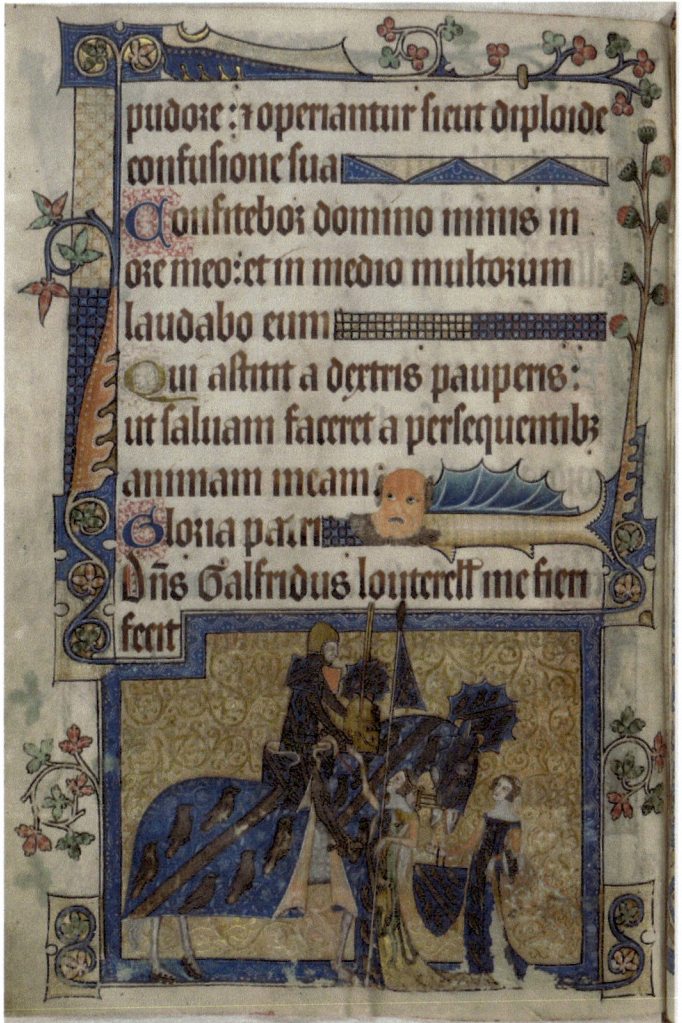

▶ A page from the Luttrell Psalter, 1320–1340

Britain 1250–1500: an overview

Record

The next four pages summarise different aspects of life in medieval England. Read through them quickly and make a list of at least six specific features that you think may have affected people's health at that time. Collect and explain your ideas in a table like this:

Specific feature of life at this time	How I think this may have affected the people's health

1. God's world and God's people

Almost everyone in medieval England was a Christian. They believed in one God who showed himself in three ways. He was:

- God the Father who made the world and ruled over all human affairs in His great wisdom. His ways were often too mysterious for human minds to grasp.
- God the Son, Jesus Christ, who came to Earth as a man and who paid for mankind's sins by dying on a cross, opening the way for believers to join God in Heaven when they died.
- God the Holy Spirit who responded to prayer and worked invisibly in people's lives, helping them to cope with suffering, to love others and to care for their needs.

While people trusted in God's goodness they also feared the power of the Devil, who constantly tried to make people doubt God's goodness.

▶ God the Father, Son and Holy Spirit from the Luttrell Psalter

2. God's Church

Every Christian was a member of God's Church. By 1250, the Roman Catholic Church in western Europe was wealthy and powerful under the leadership of the Pope and his bishops. For most people, the care of the Church came from priests who served in small areas known as parishes. By 1250, every parish in England had its own church building and many towns had beautiful cathedrals. There were also many abbeys, monasteries and convents where monks or nuns lived. They prayed for the world around them and served local people and travellers by providing food, shelter and care for those in need.

Roman Catholics believed they would not go straight to heaven when they died. Their souls first needed to suffer for a time until they had been made pure. Catholics believed they could reduce this time by doing good deeds on Earth. These included giving money and care to the sick and needy.

◀ Two nuns pray for each other and for the needs of the world. From the Luttrell Psalter

Did anyone really care about health in medieval England?

3. Kings: the servants of God

Medieval people believed that God had put kings on Earth to rule over them and keep them safe. Kings were supposed to serve God by defending the nation from its enemies, by maintaining law and order and by encouraging trade. Some did this well but a nation might suffer when its king was lazy or wasted money in wars.

Kings taxed their people and demanded certain services from them. The money from these taxes paid for the king's family and his court to live in a grand style and funded the work of some royal officials. Medieval government did far less for people than we expect today. In fact these kings had nothing like the wealth of the great Roman Empire that had ruled Britain long ago. The Romans provided their citizens with good roads, fine buildings and a good water supply and drainage. Medieval kings did not.

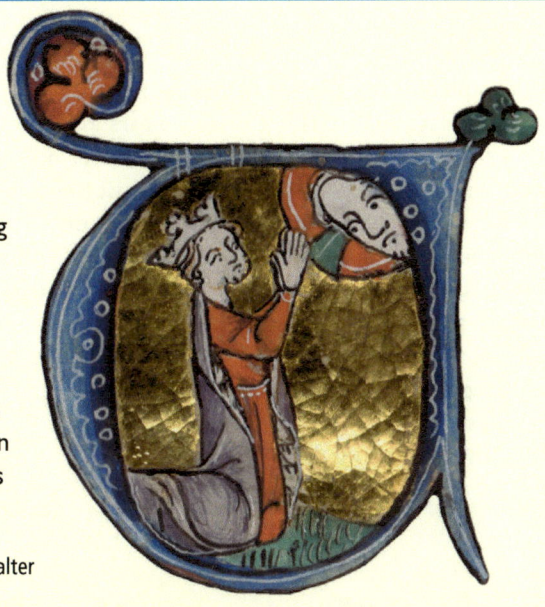

▶ A king kneels before God. From the Luttrell Psalter

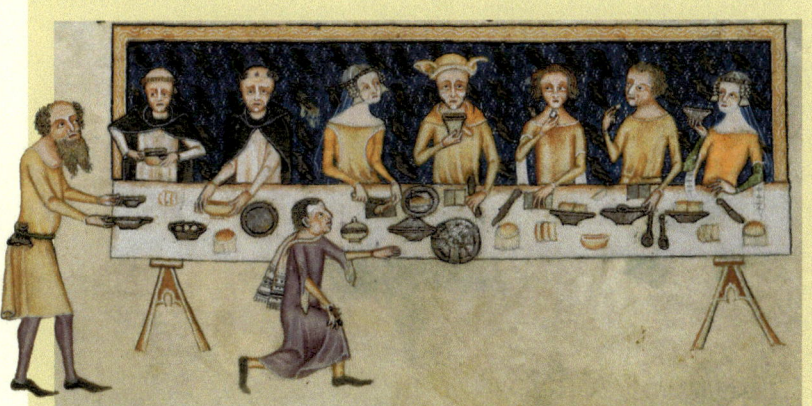

▲ Sir Geoffrey Luttrell and his family enjoy a feast. At the table with them are some priests. From the Luttrell Psalter

4. Lords: the servants of kings

The king gave land to powerful barons who, in return, controlled the different parts of the kingdom for him. The barons shared out their land amongst knights, like Sir Geoffrey Luttrell. Each parcel of land was called a manor and the knight was the lord of the manor. The farm produce from the manor allowed a knight's family to live in some comfort. All the profits went to the baron and the king. In the thirteenth century the barons and the knights won the right to sit in parliament and to have some say over what taxes the king would receive. But they still had no real control over what the king chose to do with his wealth.

5. Labourers: the servants of all

Below the king and his lords were the labourers (peasants) who did the hard, physical work that created the nation's wealth. Most served the lord of the manor by working in the fields in return for being allowed a house and some land for their own family. Others, like those serving food at the feast above, worked for wages and had no land at all. Over 90 per cent of the population lived in the countryside. Peasants knew that they could not control the world of nature. In times of bad harvest they would be the first to suffer. They had no say in how the country was ruled and their way of life depended almost completely on decisions made by the lords, the king and the Church.

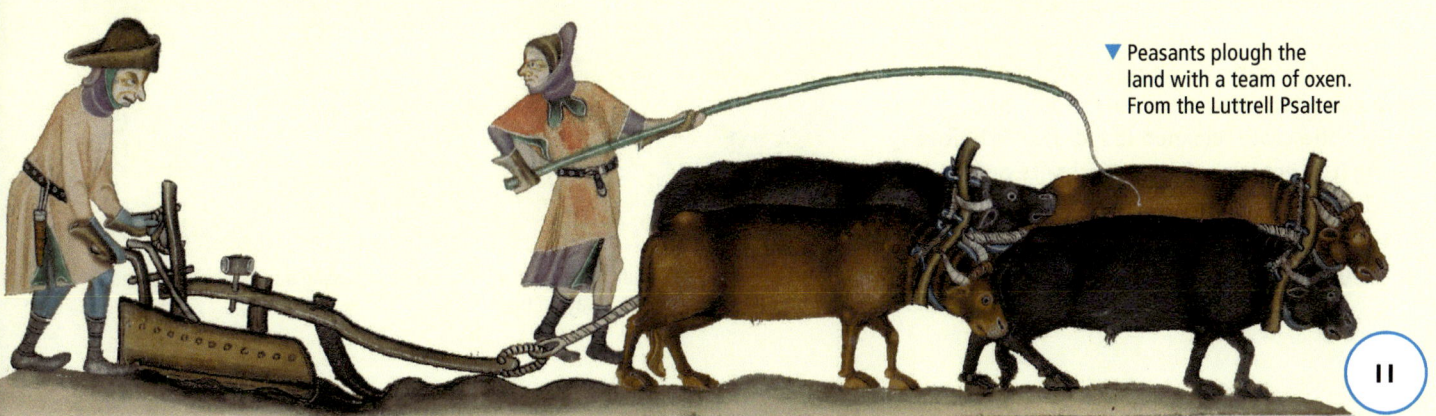

▼ Peasants plough the land with a team of oxen. From the Luttrell Psalter

6. The limits of technology

In this picture people are delivering sacks of grain to the village miller. There were no cars in medieval times and not everyone had a horse. Water mills and windmills such as this were the most powerful machinery of their day. Blades for digging or ploughing were hand-made by blacksmiths. Printing presses appeared in England from the 1470s but before then new ideas were spread by worth of mouth or handwritten text. No one had yet developed powerful lenses so microscopic creatures such as microbes and germs were completely unknown to the medieval world.

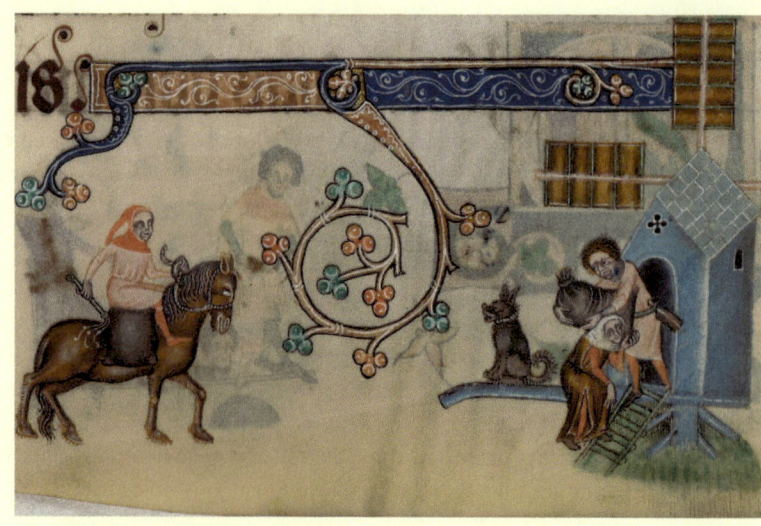

▶ A windmill, from the Luttrell Psalter.

7. The influence of ancient ideas

Some historians think that the idea for windmills, as shown above, came from Muslims who used them in their lands in Spain. The Muslims influenced medieval Europe in other ways too. Arab scholars kept alive the ideas of Greek and Roman thinkers after the fall of the Roman Empire. They wrote these down and the books made their way to Europe. The Church was happy to spread some of these ancient ideas as they matched Christian beliefs that God had made a carefully ordered Universe.

One particularly powerful idea from the Greeks said that the world was made from four elements: fire, water, air and earth. They also said that the human body was made from four liquids, or humours. These were blood, phlegm, yellow bile and black bile. The body only worked when these humours were properly balanced. Eating the right foods would balance the humours, but if a person had a fever, a doctor might cut a vein and allow blood to flow from the patient's arm so that the balance could be restored.

◀ A doctor balances a patient's humours by letting blood flow from his arm. From the Luttrell Psalter

8. The growth of the wool trade

Sheep provided milk, meat and manure but their fleece was also highly valuable. By the end of the Middle Ages, England was famous for the wool that she exported to Europe. Women would spin the raw wool into yarn that was then woven into cloth. This provided extra income for country workers and raised their standard of living, and added to the nation's wealth. But the people who gained most were wool traders who bought the cloth, cleaned it and dyed it before selling it at great profit to merchants on the continent of Europe. The wool trade added to the nation's wealth and led to the growth of many English towns.

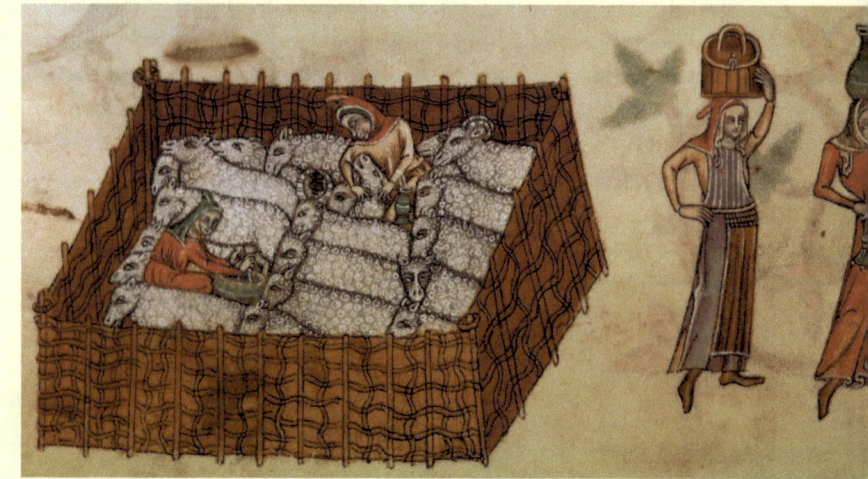

▲ A sheep pen from the Luttrell Psalter. The sheep are being inspected and milked. The women carry milk away on their heads.

Did anyone really care about health in medieval England?

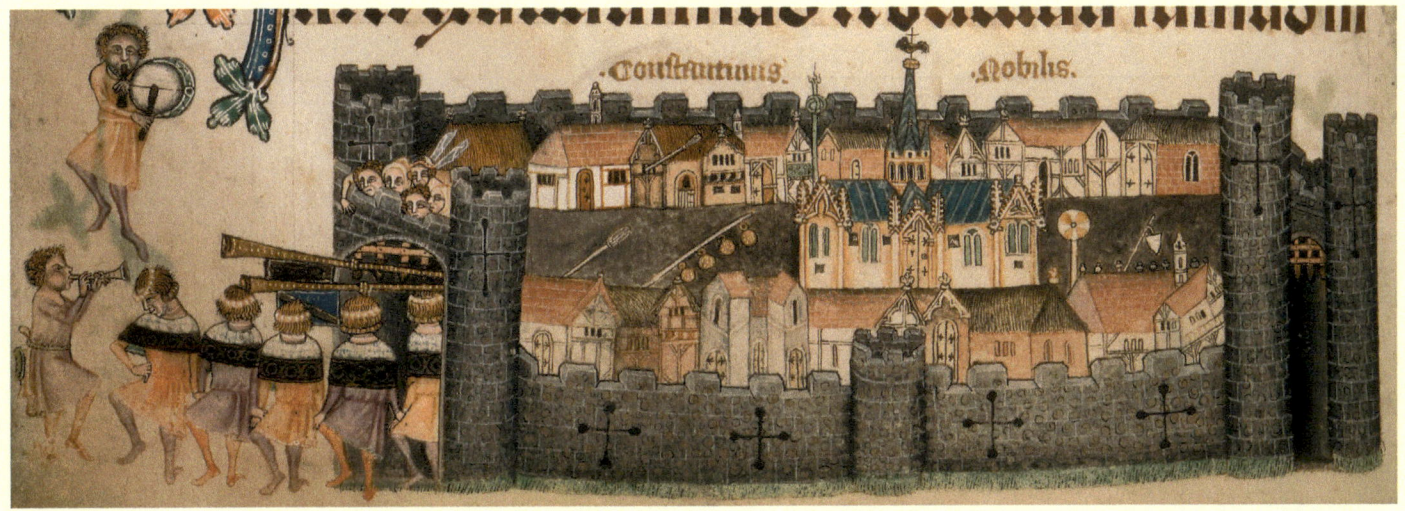

▲ A celebration in a medieval town. From the Luttrell Psalter

9. The growth of towns

Even as late as 1500, there were only about fifteen towns in England that had a population of more than 10,000. By the standards of our own day these towns were not very large, but in the Middle Ages they felt crowded and busy. They were especially crowded on market days when traders of all sorts sold their wares. Peasants from surrounding villages also came to the market to sell spare produce for cash. But even without the market, the town was full of activity, noise and mess as all sorts of craftsmen and women went about their business.

Unlike villages, towns were not controlled by lords. Instead, a mayor and a town council of important men created rules that aimed to keep law and order. They wanted their town to prosper so that everyone could be proud of it. They also made rules to keep people safe from dangers such as an outbreak of fire.

Many town councillors were also members of guilds. These were bodies that controlled the quality and price of the goods that were made in the town. There were guilds for cloth workers, bakers, brewers and all sorts of trades. The guilds were also deeply religious groups and tried hard to look after the welfare of the town community in many different ways.

10. Daily life and leisure

Medieval people enjoyed a drink, especially on the many holidays (holy days) in honour of saints. The people leaving the town gate in the image above may be celebrating one of these. But at any time a friendly drink might lead to a drunken disturbance. The two men in this picture have turned to violence and are hitting each other with clay pots that may have held their ale. By showing them with the legs of wild animals, the artist who painted this scene in the Luttrell Psalter may be suggesting that this was 'beastly' behaviour.

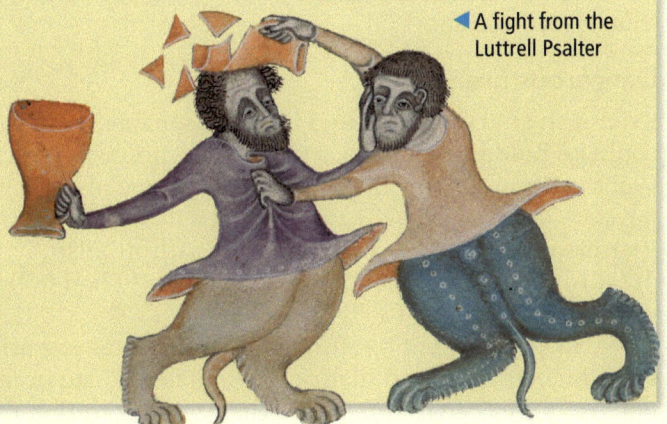

◀ A fight from the Luttrell Psalter

Record

Complete the notes in your table. At the end of your enquiry you will have the chance to see how many of your speculations about health in the Middle Ages proved to be accurate.

Living conditions

Record

By now you should have a good overview of medieval life and some ideas about how this may have affected people's health. Now we can look in more detail at the conditions in which people lived in the Middle Ages.

Our health has always depended very much on what we eat and drink, the air we breathe, the houses we live in, how clean we can keep ourselves and what we do with all the waste we create – especially the waste from our own bodies!

On the next six pages you will be reading about the living conditions of medieval people, firstly in the countryside and then in the towns. As you read, make notes in two columns like this:

Helpful for health	Hazardous for health

Life on the land: the countryside

Daily bread

On page 11 you saw peasants from the Luttrell Psalter ploughing the land. In this image they are reaping the harvest. Peasants worked hard on the land. Their lives depended on it. The woman standing up in this picture seems to have thrown away her sickle so that she can stretch out her back. But she is working in fresh air with friends and family and she would have been used to doing hard, physical work from a very young age.

Nothing mattered more than the harvest in medieval life. A good harvest gave some chance of health and comfort. A bad harvest meant a dearth of food – and dearth meant death. After years of plenty and population growth, a dreadfully wet summer and terrible harvest led to the Great Famine of 1315–16. This was followed by outbreaks of animal disease that attacked cattle and sheep. The bad weather and poor harvests lasted until 1322. The peasants were helpless against these disasters. About ten per cent of the population died in this Great Famine.

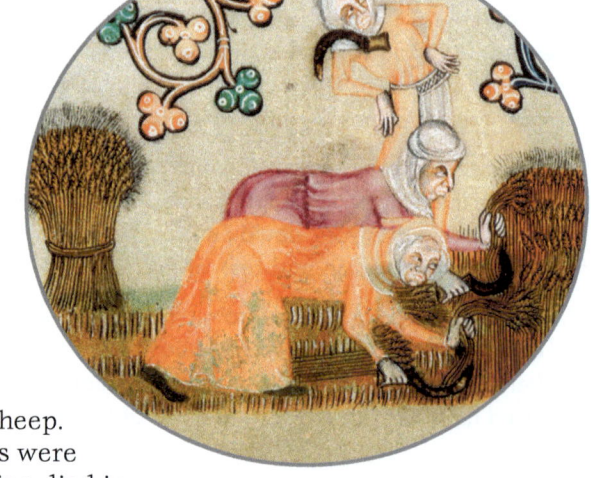

▲ Gathering the harvest, from the Luttrell Psalter, early fourteenth century

Dangerous bread

Even if the harvest appeared to be reasonable, as in the picture above, there could be hidden problems. In damp conditions, a certain fungus grew on rye, the grain used to make the type of bread eaten by people living in poverty. We now know that the fungus causes a disease called ergotism. Victims suffered from an outburst of painful pustules on their skin and a dreadful burning sensation. They frequently had hallucinations and many went mad.

No one connected the fungus with the disease until the 1670s. Then a French doctor realised that richer people who ate bread made from wheat, not rye, never caught ergotism. He also noticed that the disease only struck in years with wetter summers when the fungus grew on the rye. Only after microscopes were developed did scientists prove that the cause of this disease was the fungus on rye. Medieval people believed it was caused by demons. They named it 'St Anthony's Fire' after the Christian saint they believed might heal its unfortunate victims.

▼ A victim of St Anthony's Fire from the Isenheim Altarpiece by Matthias Grunewald, 1516

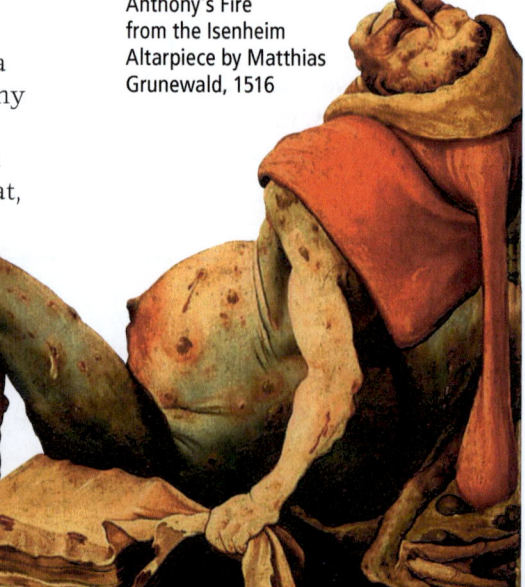

Did anyone really care about health in medieval England?

Water and drink

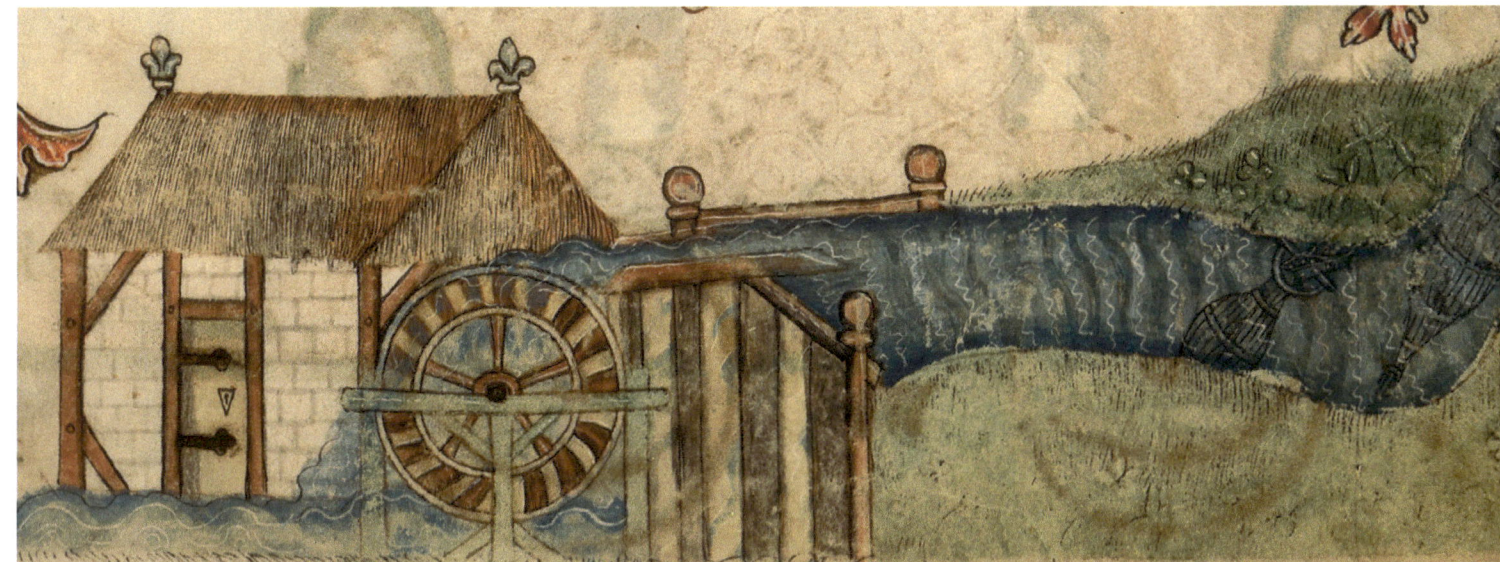

▲ A water mill, from the Luttrell Psalter

Every village was near a stream or spring that provided water for humans and their animals. Springs often fed at least one well in the village, as the water from these was cleaner than water taken from streams where animals went to drink. From records of deaths by accidental drowning, we know that peasants sometimes bathed in the streams, usually in the summer months.

> **An extract from a coroner's report covering the Oxford area**
> July 13, 1346
> John de Salesbury on Wednesday bathed in the Thames and was drowned.

Some streams turned water wheels. Most mills ground grain but in the later Middle Ages, when the textile industry had expanded into the countryside, there were many fulling mills. Fullers cleaned newly woven cloth with a mixture that was largely made up of human urine. They then softened the cloth by pounding it with mighty wooden hammers, powered by the water mill. This must have made a terrible noise. Until water mills did this job, men and women had softened the cloth by foot while it was being cleaned in the urine mixture. Fulling in the countryside polluted many streams.

If you look closely at the stream in the picture, you can see nets in the water. These are catching fish and eels. Fish is an important part of a healthy diet. Medieval people did not know that it provides important vitamins, but they did know that on Fridays fish would be the only meat that they ate. The Church insisted that no one ate meat from land animals on the day of the week when Christ had been crucified. Many villages created their own fish ponds.

Medieval villagers probably drank more water than most town dwellers, but they had other options including cider, made from the apples that grew around them, or mead, a drink made from honey. Ale brewed from barley was an important part of their diet and gave valuable nutrition. The most common ale was known as 'small beer'. This was not as strong as today's beers. It had just enough alcohol in it to stop the brew from going bad for a few days. Boiling the brew for hours also killed off any germs in the water, although no one at the time knew this.

> **Reflect**
> Which of the hazards you have recorded so far do you think were the most serious threats to people's health in the Middle Ages?

The peasants' houses

The villages had some common land where all peasants could graze their cattle and sheep. Pigs, watched by a swineherd, would search for food in the woodland nearby. Geese, ducks and hens were kept closer to the houses and often wandered inside.

The houses varied in size. The biggest belonged to the lord of the manor. Some peasants lived in very simple huts with walls woven from sticks and covered in mud. But many lived in quite large houses with strong timber frames like the one shown in this drawing.

An open wood fire on a stone hearth was used for cooking and warmth. The most common food was pottage, like a thick soup made in a large iron pot. It contained peas or beans and onions. It was eaten with bread bought from a village baker or made in the village oven that was shared by all. Sometimes animal bones were used in the pottage and you can see meat such as mutton, beef or pork hanging in the smoke-filled rafters in the picture. The smoke preserved the meat.

There was no chimney and the smoke billowed around before leaving through a hole in the thatched roof. Windows were very small with wooden shutters, not glass. Bringing the valuable cows inside the house at night kept the animals safe and the peasants warm. The floor was covered with rushes or straw. Archaeologists have found floors that have been hollowed by regular sweeping with brooms.

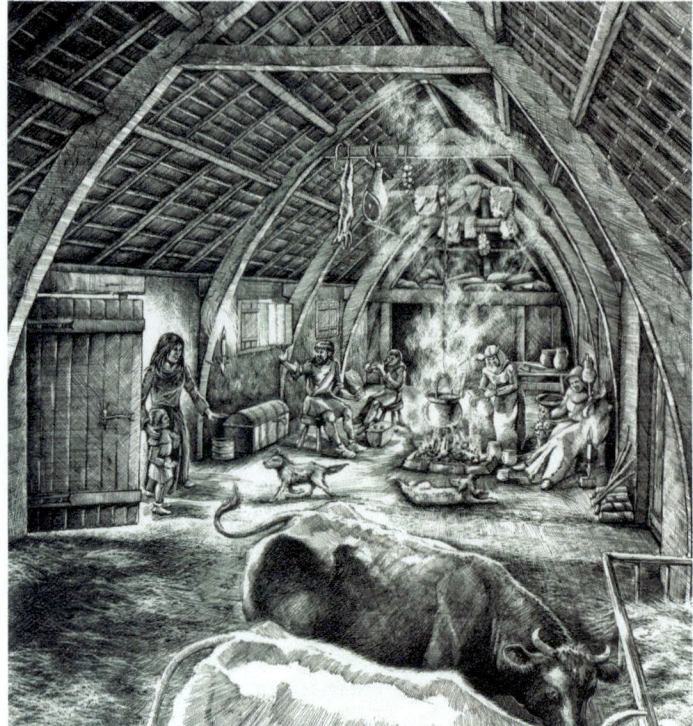

▲ An artist's reconstruction of a peasant's house, drawn c.1990

▼ Types of cesspit

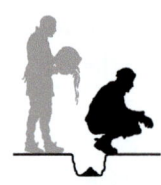

Cat hole

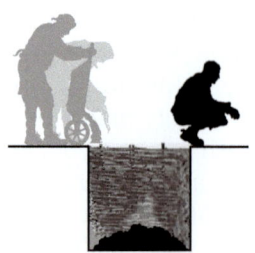

Waste pit or straddle trench

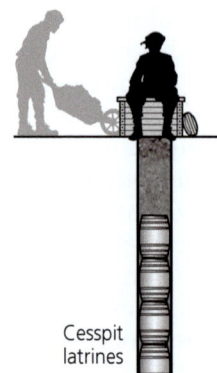

Cesspit latrines

Gardens and waste

Most village houses had a kitchen garden where peasants grew vegetables and fruit. With nuts gathered from the woods, honey from beehives, milk and cheese from cows or sheep and eggs from hens, they had a healthy diet.

In each garden was a midden or rubbish tip. Floor sweepings, waste from cooking and broken pots would all be thrown on this. So would animal droppings and possibly human excrement. Some houses had their own cesspit, but in many cases peasants probably just dug shallow holes in their gardens and squatted over them, covering the mess with ash from the fire hearth. Or they may have just taken themselves off to the nearby woods.

The waste from middens and cesspits was valuable. Every so often it was collected onto a cart and spread over the fields to fertilise the soil. Some peasants could read and had simple books on farming. These advised them how to use the manure according to the ancient Greek ideas about the four humours.

Medieval waste has been valuable to historians as well: much of what we know about the diet and lifestyle of medieval peasants comes from analysing the pips, seeds, nutshells, bones and broken pottery that can be found either where the midden once lay or out in the fields where its rubbish was spread in a mixture with straw and animal urine. The signs of large quantities of moss found in cesspits suggests how they coped in years before lavatory paper.

Record

Add some more notes to your helpful/hazardous columns.

Did anyone really care about health in medieval England?

Life in the towns

From time to time peasants would travel to their nearest town where living conditions were rather different.

Roads and streets

Peasants might use the same cart that took the rubbish from the midden to the fields to take grain, fruit, fish, cheese, timber, cloth and other goods (including fresh moss) to the towns to be sold in the market. Some carts had iron-studded wheels to give extra grip on the slippery roads. As there were no refrigerated lorries to carry butchered meat, drovers walked livestock such as cattle to town.

Country roads turned to mud in winter. In the towns, roads near the centre were often paved or cobbled and so was the market place, but these often broke up and turned back to dirt and mud. The drains down the centre of the streets were easily damaged by carts and animals.

> **Record**
> Continue your notes as you read about towns.

Markets and shops

Markets were central to town life. In the streets around the market, traders served customers from the spaces in front of their houses. In this image from fifteenth-century Italy, you can see a tailor making clothes, a barber washing and shaving a customer, and a man selling herbs and spices. The white pillar on the green tablecloth is a sugar loaf, from which some granules were scraped and sold. Sugar was a rare and expensive treat in the Middle Ages. Most people used honey to sweeten food.

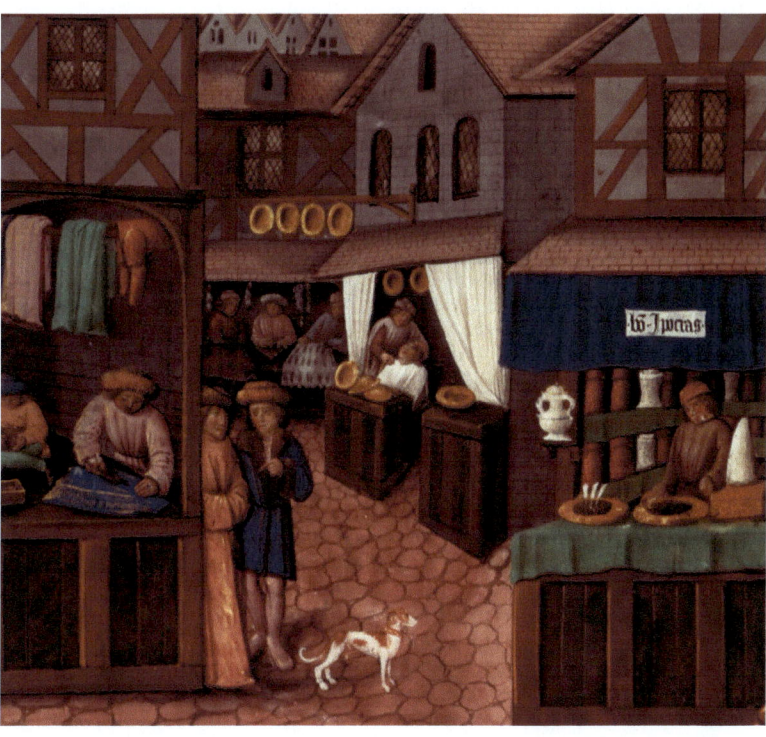

▲ Shops in a fifteenth-century Italian town

The town's water and waste

In the centre of the market square some towns had a conduit. This was a fountain where spring water flowed for all to use. The water was channelled into the town through lead pipes from springs in the countryside. The earliest conduits were built by the Church. Cathedrals and friaries in the town needed clean water for acts of worship and they could afford to lay the pipes. By the fifteenth century, as towns grew richer, the town council had often taken over the maintenance of these conduits. Water-carriers filled leather sacks at these conduits and went selling from door to door.

Street vendors and taverns sold hot food and ale. Sometimes vendors made meat pies from old or rancid meat. Tavern ale was strong brewed ale and drunkenness was a common problem, despite the Church's warnings about the sins of gluttony. For those in need, there were public latrines around many markets. In 1423, the wealthy Mayor of London, Richard Whittington, left money in his will for more latrines to be built in London.

At the end of a market day the streets were full of waste from food and other goods that had been on sale. There was also the dung dropped by all the animals. From 1293, London paid rakers to clear the streets and to dispose of the rubbish outside the town walls. From there it could be taken by the peasants and spread on the fields. By 1500, most other towns employed rakers as well.

▼ A water seller, from the Luttrell Psalter

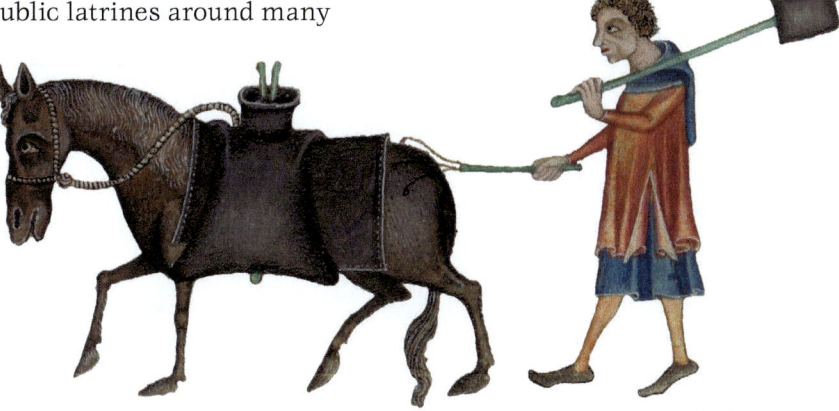

Trades and mess

Medieval trades created all sorts of pollution in the urban environment. Butchers were among the worst offenders but their work was vital as this diagram suggests.

Butchering animals made a dreadful mess. By the end of the Middle Ages most councils had ordered all butchers and fishmongers to do their cutting on the outskirts of the town and dispose of the rubbish themselves. By 1500 some towns employed carters to collect and remove waste from butchers and fishmongers. Other industries had to work on the edge of town too:

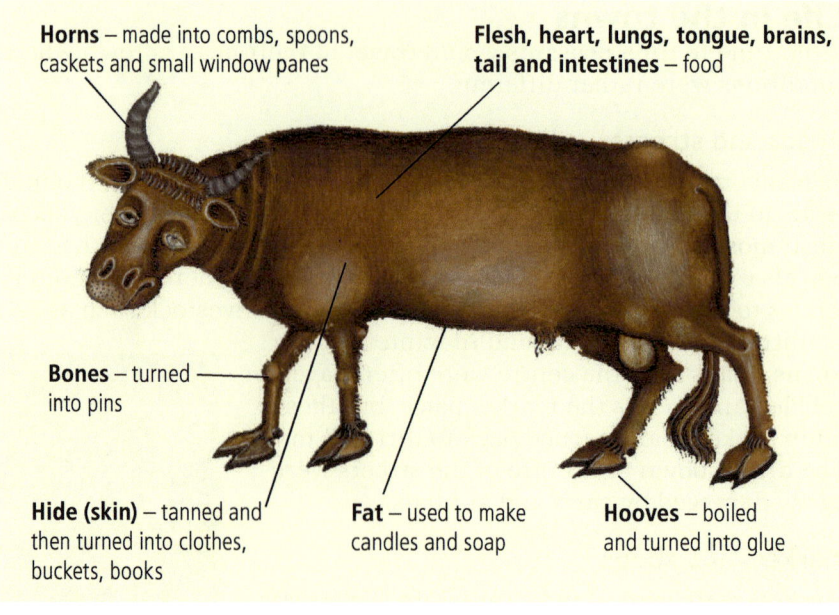

Horns – made into combs, spoons, caskets and small window panes

Flesh, heart, lungs, tongue, brains, tail and intestines – food

Bones – turned into pins

Hide (skin) – tanned and then turned into clothes, buckets, books

Fat – used to make candles and soap

Hooves – boiled and turned into glue

- Tanners scraped hair from animal hides and used natural acids to make them soft.
- Brewers were left with large deposits of barley husks after making ale that nourished people.
- Dyers needed to dispose of the liquids in which they soaked the cloth that went on to keep people warm.
- Washerwomen created large quantities of soapy water as they kept people clean by washing their clothes.
- Masons (builders) were left with rubble and dust after making and mending the houses that sheltered people.
- Lime burners made the limewash paint that stopped rainwater from destroying the walls of buildings.

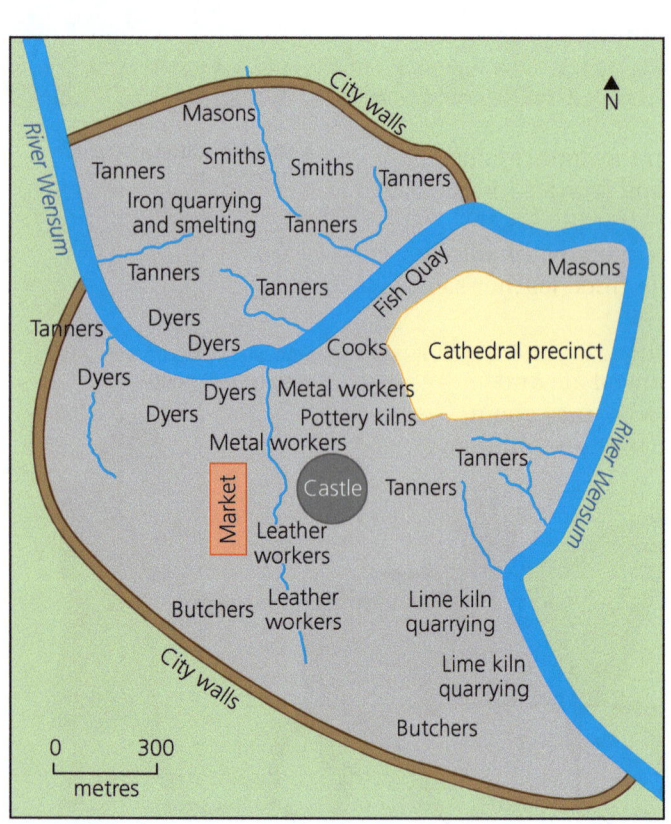

Smell

Some industries created smells as well as physical waste. Some lime burners had started to use sea-coal, which made a terrible smell. So had metal workers, such as the people who made the lead pipes that brought water into the city.

Archaeologists have compared the skeletons of children from town and countryside in the Middle Ages. Evidence from the bones around the nose shows that town children suffered from damaged sinuses, a sure sign of breathing difficulties. Children from the country did not. For people at the time, the smell was a problem for a very different reason: they believed that the main cause of disease was an invisible poison in the air. They called this poisoned air 'miasma'. A monk writing in 1240 about the ideas of Greek and Arab doctors warned that:

> **From a book written in 1240 by a monk, Bartholomaus Anglicus**
>
> If the vapour in the air is malicious, stinking and corrupt, it corrupts the spirit inside humans and often brings pestilence.

◀ Norwich in the fourteenth century, showing the locations of different trades

Did anyone really care about health in medieval England?

House and garden

Rich merchants might have owned houses like the one shown here. The upper floors jutted out to provide more floor space inside, but this shut out sunlight from the narrow streets below. In the Middle Ages it probably had a thatched roof where all sorts of insects, mice and rats would have lived.

In the centre of town, houses were tightly packed together but further out many had gardens. The occupants grew flowers believing that their scent purified the foul air that might cause disease. They also grew vegetables and kept animals such as chickens and pigs whose dung made a fine compost heap. The rich loved to eat meat and, although they consulted food guides that told them which meats might affect their humours, it cannot have been a healthy diet. Most townspeople ate similar food to villagers, but with greater variety from the market.

Householders were supposed to keep their gutters in good order and clear drains and streets around their property but not everyone did. Rainwater could go stagnant in puddles, adding to the smells that medieval people believed were dangerous. The fact that rich citizens shared the city with everyone else meant that they did what they could to limit these problems, especially in the areas where they lived.

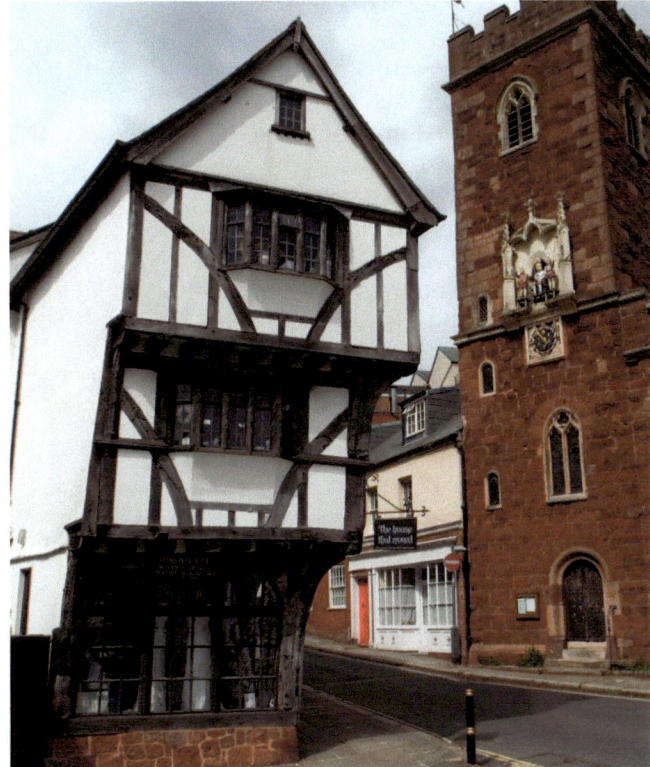

▼ A fifteenth-century merchant's house in Exeter

Water and waste

No one had pipes to bring clean water into the house. A few had their own well, but most had to collect water from the town conduit or buy it from the water carrier. People used the water for cooking, washing and brewing their own ale. If they drank water they might warm it first as this was supposed to help keep their humours in balance.

Householders were allowed to put rubbish on the street outside their houses for three or four days, but could be fined after that if they, or the rakers of the town, had not taken it away. Human waste was more of a problem. The rich might have had a latrine inside their house but for most people it was outside in a yard. Several houses might have shared a latrine. The waste dropped into a cesspit. Expensive cesspits were really well-made from stone and were watertight. Others were lined with barrels sunk into the ground. The worst latrines had no lining and the excrement would have leaked into the cellars of neighbouring houses.

When a latrine was full (or preferably before then) a professional *gongfermer* would scoop out all the mess and take it away. This might involve climbing down into the pit. The *gongfermers'* duties included taking cartloads of cess out of the town but only at night. They often sold this to farmers with land just outside the walls, but some simply tipped it into nearby streams like the one outside Exeter called Shitbrook.

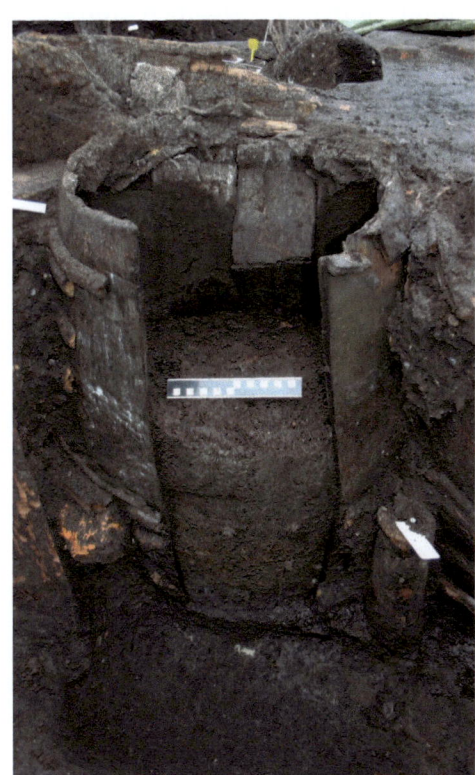

▲ A barrel used to line a cesspit. This one is from an archaeological dig in Denmark but similar ones have been found in English towns. Archaeologists have cut away the side to reveal the thirteenth-century contents still inside.

Record

Finish your notes on things that helped health or were hazards to health. Highlight the three most important discoveries you made.

Responses to the Black Death

Deadly epidemics were a familiar part of life in the Middle Ages, especially in times of famine. Some of these epidemics were associated with poor food or dirty living conditions. These included ergotism, typhoid and dysentery (severe diarrhoea), but none of these compared with the most dreadful killer disease in human history: plague.

Rumours about a terrifying disease from the east reached England late in 1347. By then it had struck Sicily in southern Europe. People in England assumed that it would never reach them. But it did and it killed millions. It has become known as the 'Black Death'.

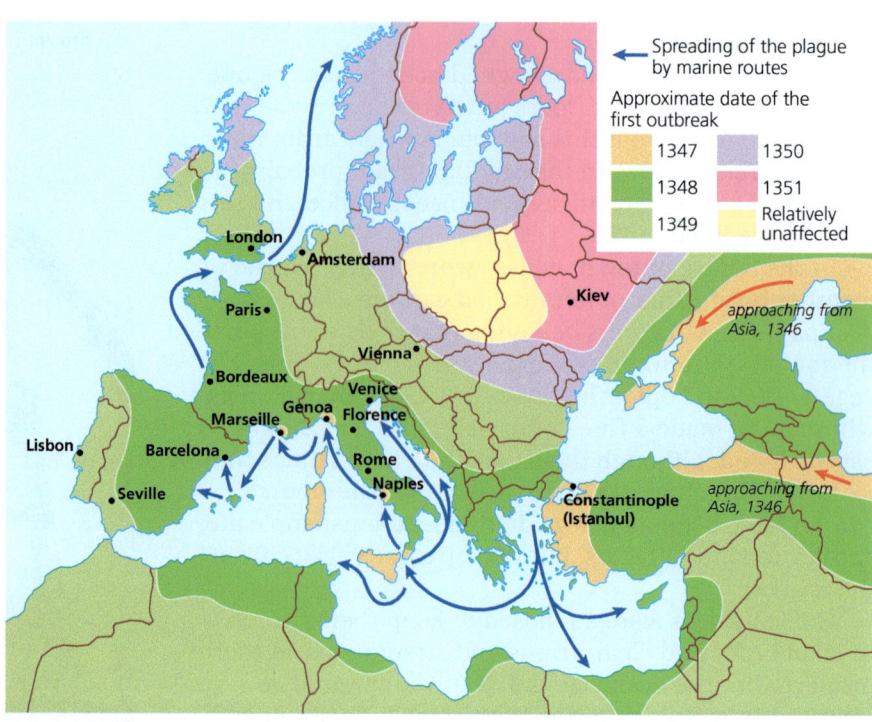

▲ Map showing the movement of the Black Death, or plague, into and through Europe

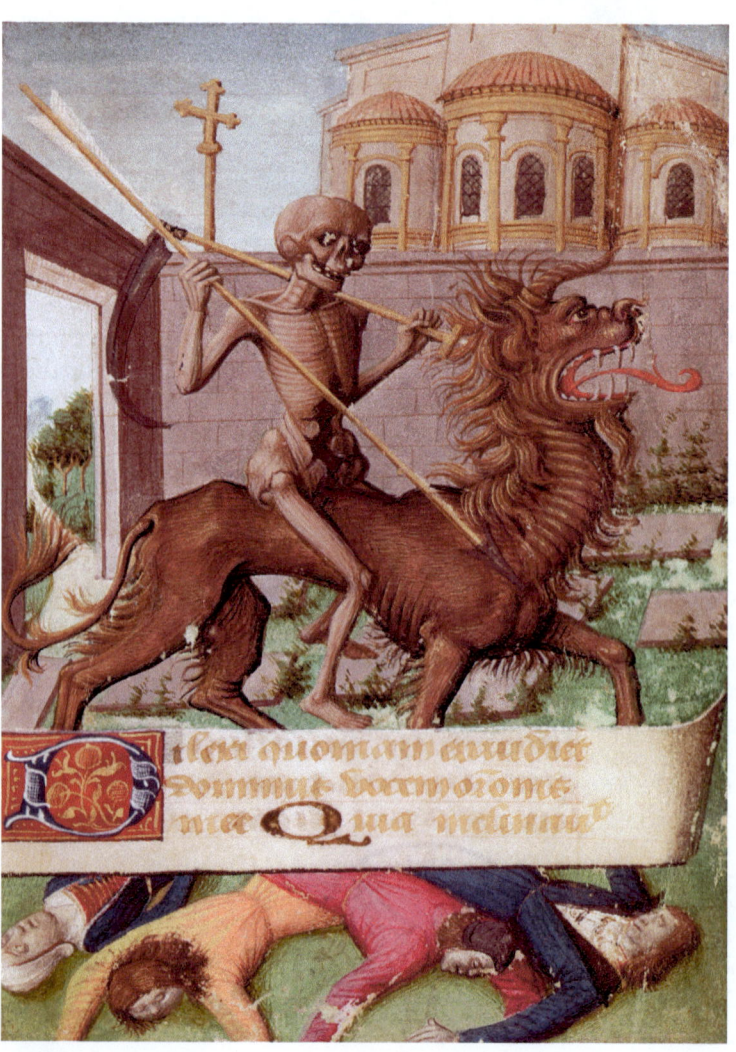

Arrival and spread

The plague first reached England in the summer of 1348 at Melcombe, a port in Dorset. Within weeks it had struck Bristol and London. No one was safe, whether in town or country, rich or poor. It could not be stopped. By the end of 1349 it had spread to the far north of England, to all of Wales and into Ireland.

Plague is caused by a bacillus or germ called *Yersinia pestis*. The germ lives in the guts of fleas. When a flea bites its victim it regurgitates the germ and spreads the infection. The disease started in Asia and reached Europe along the trade routes from east to west. Fleas liked to live on black rats that infested the trading ships that sailed between Europe's ports. The rats came ashore in harbours and the disease then swiftly spread inland, carried by fleas on the rats or in the clothing of human hosts. Today, plague can be treated with antibiotics, but these were only discovered in the twentieth century. Medieval people knew nothing about plague's link with rats and fleas, and did not even know that germs existed.

◀ The figure of Death as a skeleton, from a French prayer book, 1350. He rides a strange lion and strikes his selected victims with a spear or scythe. Death was gathering his harvest, cutting people down when their time was ripe.

Did anyone really care about health in medieval England?

Horror and helplessness

> ### Record
>
> Medieval people knew many hardships but until 1348 they had never faced anything quite like the Black Death. As you read the following three pages make notes using a table like the one below. In the column about how people responded, note their thoughts and feelings as well as any actions they took.
>
> | The Black Death in England, 1348–1350 | |
> |---|---|
> | How people responded to the Black Death (i.e. what they felt and did) | Why they did this |
> | | |

Terrifying suffering

We can sense the terror brought by the plague and learn something about its symptoms in this account by Iewan Gethin, a Welsh poet who saw for himself the effects of the disease in 1349:

> We see death coming into our midst like black smoke, a plague which cuts off the young, a rootless phantom which has no mercy for fair countenance. Woe is me of the shilling [swelling] of the armpit, seething terrible wherever it may come … It is of the form of an apple, like the head of an onion, a small boil that spares no one. Great is its seething, like a burning cinder, a grievous thing of ashy colour.

We now think that plague took three different forms.

1. **Bubonic plague**, from a flea bite, causes painful swellings (buboes) in the armpits and groin, an intense fever and blisters over the body. Death follows after just a few days.
2. **Septicemic plague** is caused when the infection reaches the bloodstream. There are no buboes but the victim bleeds freely and the fingers, toes or nose turn black and begin to rot away.
3. **Pneumonic plague** is caught by breathing in cough droplets from someone who is already infected by plague. The victim violently coughs up blood and may be dead within two days.

There was no cure for the plague but many treatments were tried. From centuries of experience, medieval people knew that camomile lotion, made from plants like daisies, offered some relief from inflammation of the skin. They applied it to the buboes and this may have eased the pain a little. (Camomile is a common ingredient in modern medicines too.) Some people tied live toads or chickens over the buboes, probably in an attempt to warm and soften the painfully hard swellings. Letting blood flow from an opened vein was a common medieval treatment for any illness involving a fever. It aimed to restore the balance of the four humours but almost certainly made the patient even weaker. Whatever they tried, nothing could save the victim of plague. It is no surprise that the number of wills made in London in 1348 was fifteen times higher than it had been in 1347.

> ### Reflect
>
> Which type of plague do you think Iewan Gethin had seen?

God's punishment

People's experience of the symptoms of plague led them to try the treatments you have just read about. Their beliefs about the causes of plague also shaped their responses.

To the medieval mind, everything that happened in this world depended on the will of God. If the plague struck a nation, town or village God was punishing them or allowing the Devil to test their faith. In this sense people believed that it was God who caused or allowed the plague. So, when a person fell ill, his or her friends and family prayed for healing. They might pray in their own words in their own homes or ask a priest to pray for them in the church with a lighted candle. In 1349 so many candles were burned that the price of wax soared. In some rare cases individuals did recover. But why God saved some and not others was a mystery that was beyond them.

People did all they could to persuade God to spare them from the plague so that it would miss them altogether:

- Priests urged everyone to confess their sins and to promise to mend their ways.
- At special church services people ate holy bread, blessed by the priest.
- The king ordered bishops to arrange large processions of priests through cities, confessing the nation's sins and praying that the plague would disappear.
- Groups of flagellants came to England from northern Europe. They walked in line, whipping the bare back of the person ahead of them with leather thongs that had sharp pins knotted in them. They were suffering on behalf of others and believed that God would take away the plague when he saw their love and self-sacrifice. Very few English people copied them.

Even though medieval people believed that God caused or allowed the plague to sweep the world, they tried to understand how plague killed its victims, often following theories passed down from the ancient Greeks and Romans. Some of their ideas are summarised below. These may help to explain some of the treatments you read about on page 21.

- Many claimed that unusual movements of the planets started the plague. Others blamed earthquakes in distant lands.
- Most people believed that plague infected its victims through miasma, an invisible poison in the air. This miasma was most likely to be present when the air smelled bad or where sins were committed.
- People carried posies of flowers or burned rosemary and other sweetly scented plants to purify the air in their houses.
- They believed miasma could infect people through sweaty skin so it was dangerous to take hot baths or do vigorous exercise.
- Others claimed that it was possible to catch the disease by looking a plague victim in the eye, so they turned their heads away from those who were suffering.
- The people most vulnerable to the disease were those whose humours were out of balance, often caused by eating a poor diet.

From a sermon by the Bishop of Winchester in October 1348

It is not within the power of man to understand God's plan. But it is to be feared that the most likely explanation is that human sensuality ... has now plumbed greater depths of evil ... provoking God's anger.

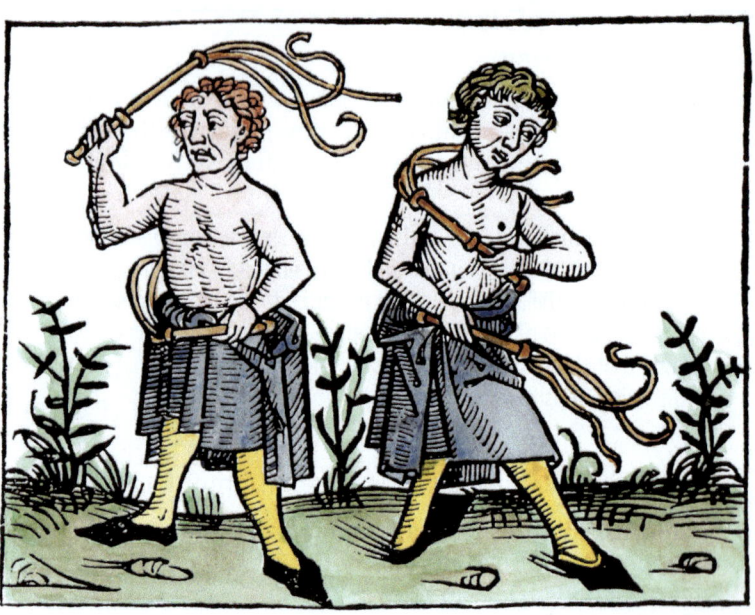

▲ Flagellants shown in a fifteenth-century woodcut

Reflect

1. Why might people have believed that a miasma caused the plague?
2. Why might people have believed that they could catch the plague by simply looking a victim in the eye?

Did anyone really care about health in medieval England?

Overwhelming impact

No matter what medieval people did to protect themselves, this Great Pestilence could not be stopped. It travelled five hundred miles in five hundred days, reaching the far north of England by December 1349. Historians used to believe that it killed about one third of England's population but recent research suggests that the figure may have reached sixty per cent. If so, 3.5 million people died in two years.

The death toll disrupted normal life. Priests were supposed to offer the 'last rites' to dying victims but they could not keep up and the Church authorities relaxed this rule. In towns, the churches no longer offered individual funerals and buried bodies in mass graves. Some priests were scared to visit the sick and lead funerals beside evil smelling graves. They simply ran away from their parishes.

The plague hit especially hard in the towns. It spread rapidly from house to house. Householders forced lodgers and even children onto the streets if they showed any signs of sickness. The rich often moved to the countryside, hoping to find pure air. Others just shut themselves away, throwing waste onto the streets. In rare cases they even threw out the bodies of plague victims. It became harder than ever to clear the mess.

In April 1349, King Edward III wrote a letter to the Mayor of London with explicit instructions to clean up the city.

> **From a letter from King Edward III to the Mayor of London in 1349**
>
> ... cause the human faeces and other filth lying in the streets and lanes to be removed with all speed to places far distant ... and to cause the city and suburbs to be cleansed from all odour and to be kept clean as it used to be in the time of preceding mayors so that no greater cause of mortality may arise from such smells.

Reflect

Does this letter from King Edward suggest that London was always filthy?

Other than writing letters such as this, the King and his government did little to deal with the crisis. In Italy many towns had complete control over their own affairs. When the plague struck, they quickly passed laws to control the movement of people and goods and arranged for extra cleaning of streets and sewers. No laws like these were passed in England until the sixteenth century.

Constant threat

The Black Death in England died down during 1350. But plague had come to stay. It struck again in 1361–62 and there were twenty more outbreaks before 1500. While people still believed that it came as God's punishment for sin, the intense shock of the original Black Death was replaced by a more general and continuous fear of plague. Skeletons representing death appeared often in paintings, on tombstones and even in jewellery of the time.

After 1400 plague was restricted mainly to the towns. As we will see, this encouraged mayors and councils to take more care to keep the towns clean and to deal with anything that might create deadly miasma or upset the balance of the four humours. But it was not easy.

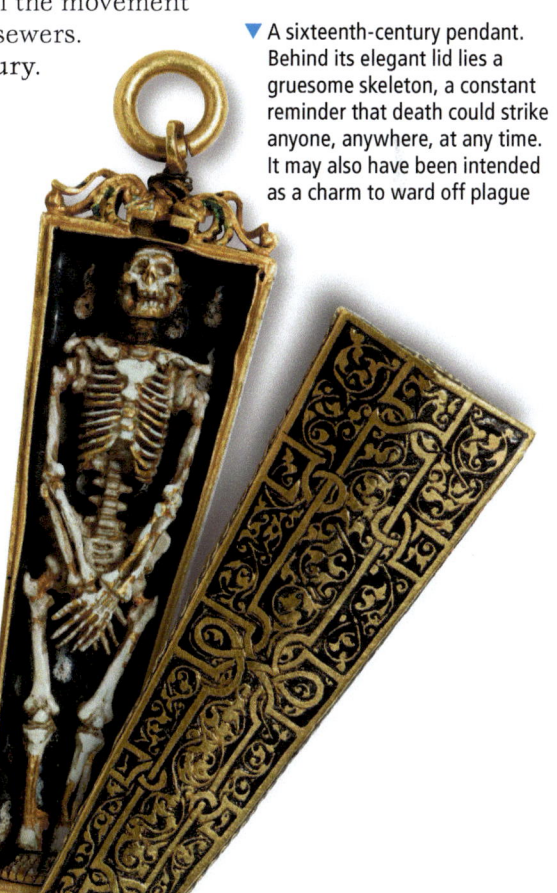

▼ A sixteenth-century pendant. Behind its elegant lid lies a gruesome skeleton, a constant reminder that death could strike anyone, anywhere, at any time. It may also have been intended as a charm to ward off plague

Record

Finish your notes on the Black Death in England. In the right-hand column, place a tick next to the three responses that you think show most clearly that medieval people really did care about keeping healthy. Place a cross against the three responses that show that medieval people did not really care about keeping healthy. Underneath your notes explain your choices.

Public health in towns and monasteries

Church authorities and health

In the thirteenth century, the church set the highest standards in hygiene. This artist's reconstruction of Fountains Abbey in Yorkshire shows the church and other buildings that provided for the needs of the 120 monks and 150 helpers who lived at the abbey. At the top right of the picture is the infirmary for the sick. Near the bottom right a block of latrines sits alongside the river whose waters flushed away the waste. Pure spring water from the hills was piped into the kitchens and to washing areas.

Smaller church communities such as cathedrals, friaries and convents needed pure water for the same reasons as large monasteries:

- It was blessed and used in baptisms and other services.
- It was mixed with wine that monks sipped during Mass.
- It was used to wash silver cups after Mass.
- It was used to wash sacred linen altar cloths.
- It was used by monks and nuns for regular washing and for baths between four and twelve times a year.
- It provided drinking and washing water as well as baths for sick townspeople who were treated by the monks and nuns.

Bringing water over long distances was expensive, especially if it involved digging trenches in the streets or in private gardens to lay pipes. Individuals could not afford to do this and few town councils had the money or desire to provide water for townspeople until the fourteenth century. A cathedral, on the other hand, had the necessary wealth, power and need. It often owned enough land in town centres to bring the pipes through its own property. This is why so many of the first town conduits were simply a short extension from the main pipe that provided the cathedral or abbey with its fresh water.

By 1500 this was changing. Standards in many monasteries had dropped while some towns were both richer and more willing to spend money on the health and hygiene of their people. As respect for the Church faded, wealthy citizens were less likely to make donations to the Church in their wills. Instead they tried to win the approval of God and the gratitude of their town by funding new conduits or public privies.

▼ An artist's reconstruction of Fountains Abbey as it may have been c.1250. Drawn by Alan Sorell, c.1967

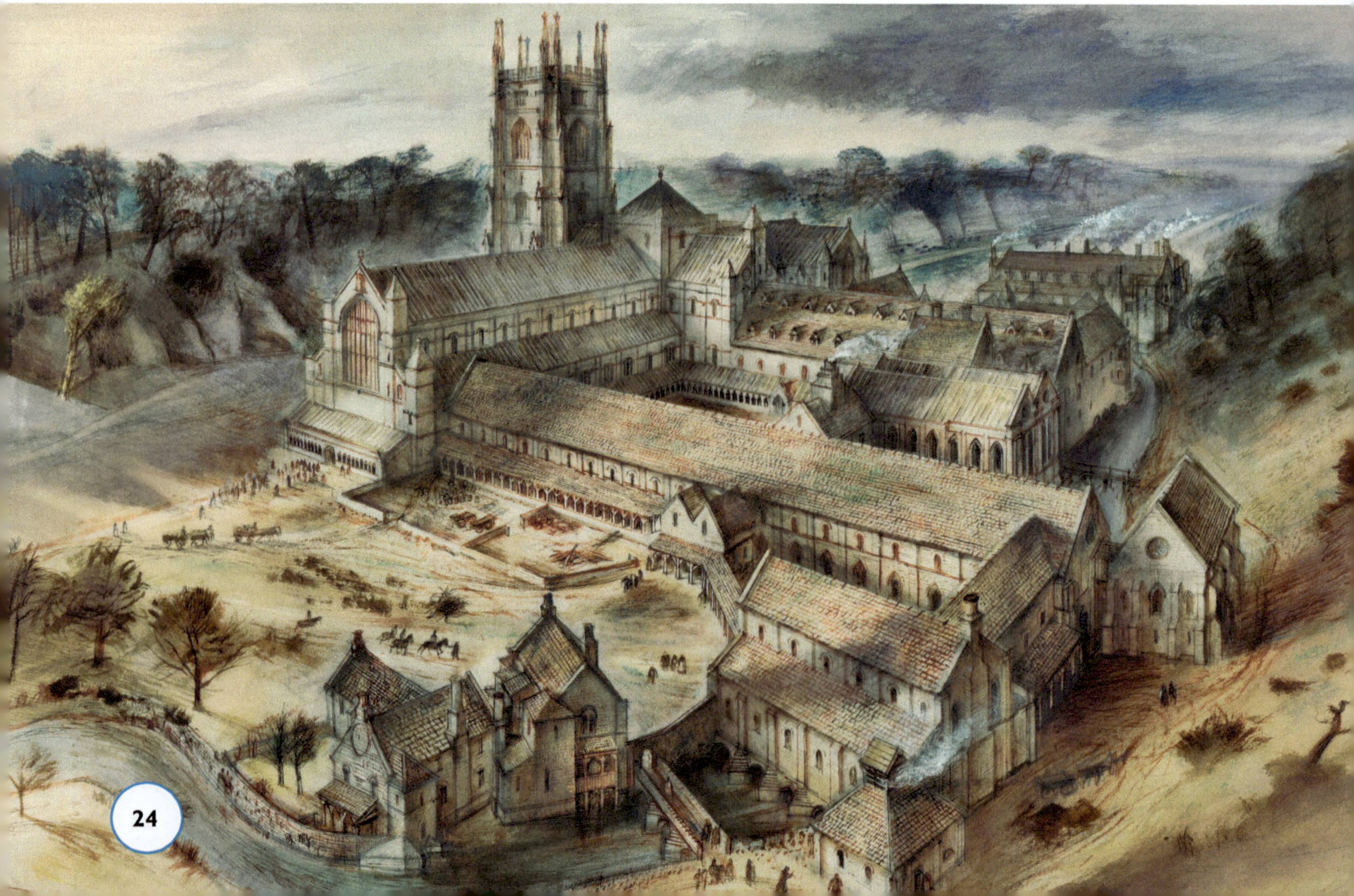

Did anyone really care about health in medieval England?

Town authorities and health

There is no doubt that medieval towns could be dirty and unhealthy, especially if we judge them by standards of our day. This is clear from records kept from the Middle Ages like the one shown here. But the records also show the efforts that towns made to deal with these problems.

The diagram below uses six towns across England to show examples of how town authorities tried to improve the environment between 1250 and 1348. On the next page you will see examples of how London tackled public health from 1348 to 1500. Read all the examples carefully and remember to follow the instructions on page 21.

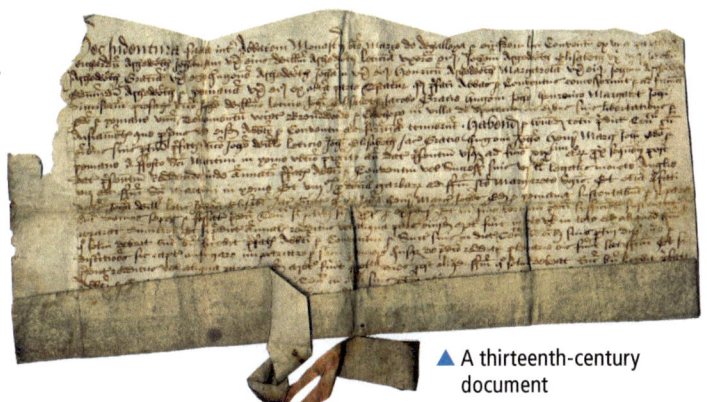

▲ A thirteenth-century document

Public health care in six English towns, 1250 to 1348

Carlisle
In 1345, officials of King Edward III reported that the streets of Carlisle were filled with dungheaps and other filth that corrupted the air. The town could not afford to clear the mess as its trade was ruined by constant attacks by Scottish raiders. To make matters worse, many dreadful diseases killed its livestock.

Shrewsbury
In 1276, King Edward I gave Shrewsbury permission to raise money from its wealthier citizens to pave the town's market place. Without paving, roads and markets were a mixture of mud, rubbish and animal dung. In his reign from 1272 to 1307, Edward I made similar arrangements in over fifty towns. He did not have enough money to pay for this work himself, but he encouraged towns to pave streets as he knew it would improve trade. If trade improved so would his income from taxes!

Bristol
In the fourteenth century, Bristol's councillors passed many by-laws. Some of these aimed to make the town more pure by moving the following to its outskirts:

- **Dungheaps**: these caused smells which, people believed, caused miasma and disease.
- **Lepers**: their breath was believed to corrupt the air and cause miasma.
- **Prostitutes**: they were sinful, and sin caused miasma.

York
In 1301, King Edward I ordered the authorities in York to clear the filth from its streets and to introduce new rules to keep the town clean. He used York as his own base in the north while he fought wars against the Scots. If the town leaders of York had ignored him they would have been in serious trouble.

Norwich
Between 1287 and 1289, sixteen citizens of Norwich were publicly named and shamed by the town's courts for polluting waterways or dumping waste. By this time, medical books were popular among the wealthy elite in England. These spread the ideas of Greek and Arab doctors about miasma. As the wealthy lived in the town with others, they had a good reason for trying to stop filth and smells building up. The town centre, where wealthy councillors lived, was usually cleaner with better drains than the outskirts, where people living in poverty had their houses.

Winchester
In 1329, the butchers' guild of Winchester appointed two people to check the quality of all meat before it could be sold. Guilds had full authority over their own trades in the town. They used set standards and made sure all guild members kept them. Guilds of food producers took this especially seriously: this kept the trust of their customers. Some guilds ordered all members to pay a fine if any one of them let quality slip. This meant everyone watched each other for any sign that standards were dropping.

Reflect

All the examples on this page are taken from the century before the Black Death struck England. If someone told you that towns only took their communities' health seriously after the Black Death arrived, what would you say?

Public health care in London, 1348 to 1500

London led the way in public health care in England. It had provided piped spring water to its citizens ever since the 1230s. It was probably the first town in the west of Europe to do this. But, despite the Black Death, its population grew from about 25,000 in 1250 to almost 100,000 in 1500. The city was crowded and dirty. It was the duty of the Lord Mayor and aldermen to run London's affairs. Many of these wealthy leaders were members of guilds that also played their part in keeping the city healthy.

> **Reflect**
>
> All the examples below about London are from the years after the Black Death when the plague returned regularly every few years. What signs can you see that this affected London's care for the health of its people?

1351	A specialist jury of London cooks found a vendor guilty of selling 'putrid and stinking' chicken pies. Specialist juries became more common as they could give an expert opinion on whether the accused person was guilty. The evil-smelling, maggot-ridden meat was burned in front of those found guilty.
1381	A specialist jury of cooks and fishmongers inspected a whole cargo of herring that had been brought up the River Thames. They found it to be 'putrid and corrupt'.
1385	A warden was appointed to check whether London's streets and the banks of the Thames were clear of 'filth and dunghills'.
1393	London's authorities built a jetty out into the Thames so that carcasses could always be carried away by boat. Butchers faced huge fines if they used other methods of disposal.
1415	The Mayor of London ordered the rebuilding of a latrine near Moorgate. It had been flooding neighbouring properties and causing sickness 'by corrupting the air'. London had set out rules about the positioning of latrines at the end of the twelfth century, but they were hard to enforce as the population grew.
1417	In this plague year, London temporarily closed the 'stews' or public baths. These baths also served as brothels. People still believed that hot baths let miasma into the body and that sin such as prostitution caused miasma to appear.
1419	London recorded all its regulations about keeping the people healthy in a special White Book because plague had killed many of the older officials who knew the ancient rules that had never before been written down.
1421	Jurors at Farringdon in London found a trader called William ate Wood (Atwood) guilty of throwing so much 'odious and infectious filth' onto the highway that people were leaving the local shops.
1430s	The Mayor of London, John Wells, organised the replacement and extension of the pipes that supplied London with fresh spring water. He and other rich citizens also gave money to the city in their wills to improve water supplies and to build new public latrines. They hoped to impress God and their fellow Londoners.
1478	London expelled tawyers (animal skinners) from the city for dumping waste into the Thames. This just moved the problem to the suburbs that were already in a worse condition than London itself.
1479	The *gongfermers* and *paviours* of London formed their own guild. London had employed professionals to repair road surfaces and clean cesspits since 1302. *Gongfermers* could earn very good pay!
1488	After Londoners called for all butchery to be banned from the city the butchers' guild built a very expensive underground passage to carry waste from the shambles (where animals were slaughtered) to the River Thames.

Did anyone really care about health in medieval England?

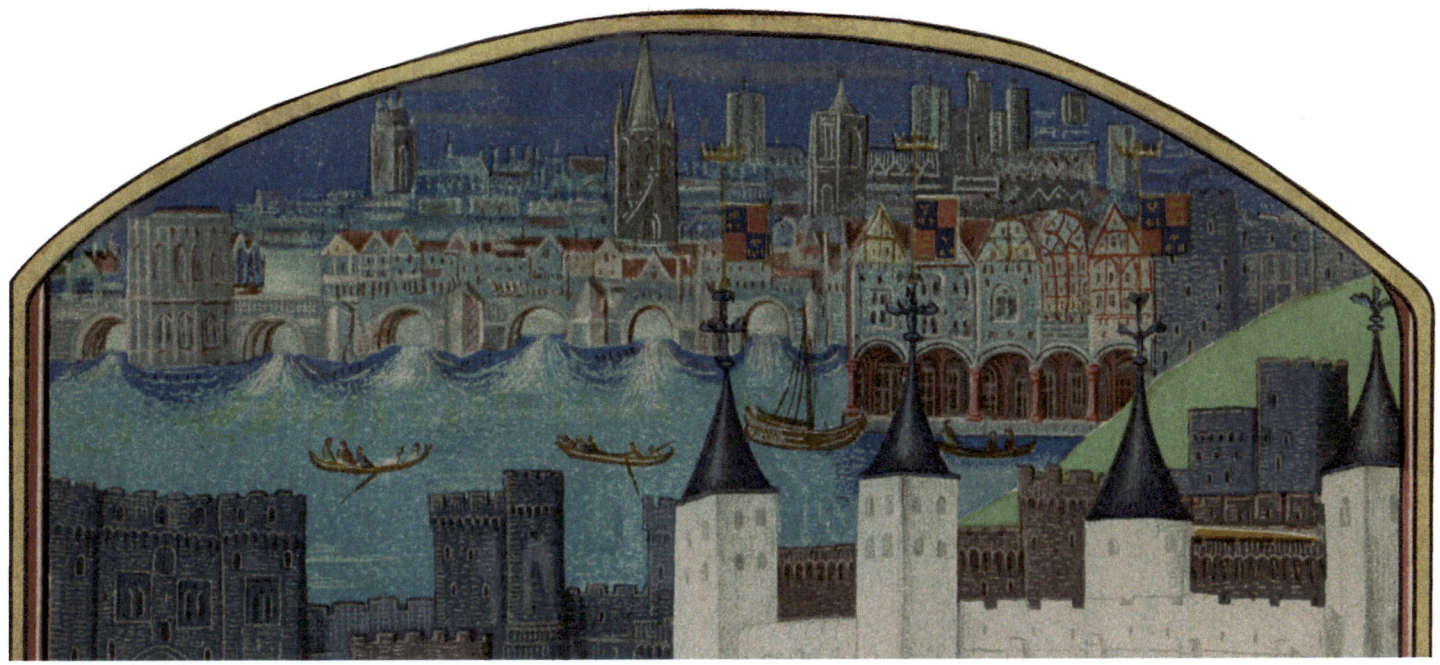

▲ London in the late fifteenth century. A detail from a sixteenth-century book of poems

Record

This task will help you to review what you have learned about public health care in medieval towns, including cathedrals.

Imagine that a web designer has asked an artist to draw a panoramic view of an imaginary medieval town. The artwork must show life going on in the town and should include twelve details that reveal interesting and important aspects of public health care. When a pointer hovers over each of these scenes a textbox will appear that explains what this detail shows about public health and what the town or church authorities were doing to try to keep people healthy.

Your job is to write a clear brief for the artist. Choose twelve aspects of health care from pages 24 to 26 that will give a good summary of what you have learned about public health in church communities and in towns. For each one, explain what the artist will need to draw and what its textbox will say when it appears on screen.

Review

A. At the start of this enquiry you listed at least six features of medieval life and explained how you thought they might have affected the people's health. Go back to that chart and review what you wrote in the light of what you have learned since then. Add some more examples and explanations of how features of medieval life mentioned in the overview on pages 10 to 13 affected the people's health.

B. The big question for this enquiry asked whether anyone really cared about health in the Middle Ages. Imagine that someone tells you that medieval people were stupid and uncaring for not looking after their health. Use what you have learned in this enquiry to write a clear, organised and well-supported reply.

CLOSER LOOK 1

Exeter's medieval water supplies

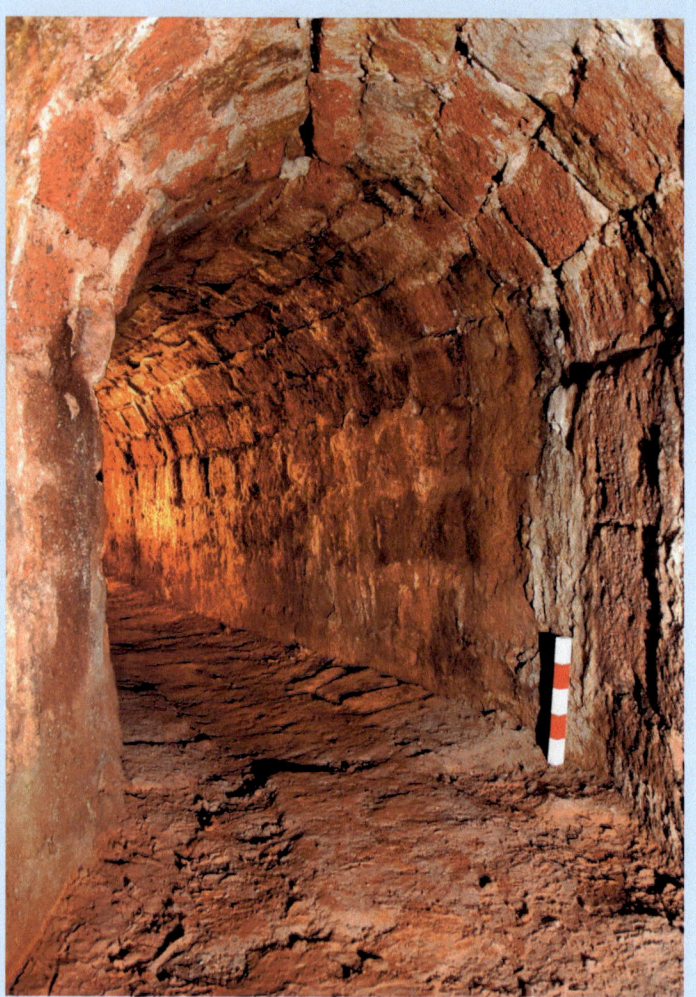

▲ A section of Exeter's fourteenth-century underground passages

Exeter in Devon provides a wonderful insight into the efforts made by medieval people to ensure they had a constant and reliable supply of pure water. Beneath the city streets are underground passages like the one shown here. They are never more than 1.5 metres high, but despite this tourists walk through them on a daily basis. Their original purpose, however, was to carry water through the city.

The water did not fill the passage itself. It flowed through lead pipes that once lay in the centre of the floor. The point of the passage was to allow workers access to the lead pipes so that they could easily carry out maintenance and repairs.

The development of this ingenious system reflects the changes in medieval life that you have just been reading about. Church records show that **by 1180** the monks at the cathedral had brought piped water into the town from a spring in the hills about a mile away to the north east. The pipes supplied both the cathedral and a smaller priory with the water they needed for holy rituals and for day-to-day washing and cooking. Another section of pipe ran to the main crossroads in the town centre. From there the townspeople could collect water for their own use. The pipe was quite small, about 8 centimetres in diameter, so there would be constant, but not spectacular, flow.

At that time there were no underground passages. The lead pipes were simply placed in ditches below ground level and covered over. When leaks occurred, which must have happened quite often, the pipe could easily be dug up and repaired.

Around the 1240s, however, the cathedral seems to have tried a new approach to laying the pipe at the point where it passed through the thick town walls. If a leak had occurred within the wall it would have been very difficult and very costly to repair. Someone had the idea of making a passage or vault through most of the thickness of the wall that could be accessed from inside the town. This meant that the pipe could be reached for maintenance very easily without needing to dig away a whole section of the wall each time.

In the 1340s really serious developments took place. This medieval parchment roll contains records of payments made by the Church for the construction of a lengthy underground passage to carry the lead pipe from the point where it came through the wall to the cathedral itself. The photograph at the top of this page shows a section of that fourteenth-century passage. In a few places, vertical shafts rise up from the main pipe. Some of these carried pipes up to ground level to feed the fountains or conduits at street level and others provided access for workers who used footholds in the stonework as a sort of ladder to climb up and down.

The records show that this passage was being finished in 1349, just as the Black Death struck Exeter.

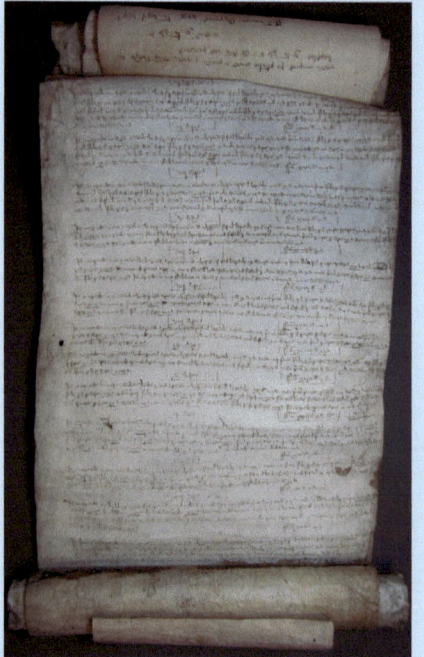

◀ Fourteenth-century church records from Exeter cathedral

The next main phase of building came **in the 1420s**. This time, the work was organised and paid for by the town council, not the Church. Exeter's wool trade helped it to grow in population and wealth in the fifteenth century. Two rich ex-mayors left money in their wills specifically to improve the town's water supply. The records tell us the name of the man who was in charge of the work. It was written as 'John Dale, plommer'. His apprentice was a boy named John Frende. Two new street level conduits were built for the people to use.

In the 1440s further improvements were made. This time the cathedral and the town council helped to fund the work, but it was definitely the town council who were in charge. This shows English towns were gaining influence and wealth, and the Church was gradually losing some of its own prestige and power. The town must have been doing well as it hired the services of an expert plumber from London. After he finished extending and improving the passages he left, but in the 1450s the town was rich enough to employ its own full-time plumber: John Frende who had worked as apprentice to John Dale thirty years before.

The town's water supply was clearly a matter of some pride. When King Henry VI visited Exeter in 1451, the great conduit at the main crossroads was chosen as the centre of the celebrations. Someone – probably John Frende – even set up two small temporary fountains and made them flow with wine throughout the king's visit.

By 1500, at the end of the Middle Ages, Exeter was once again extending its underground passageways to secure its water supply. This time the work took place outside the city walls. The aim was to lay the pipe in a passage below the main bridge that led into the east gateway. This was the route to and from London and it would help Exeter's trade if workmen could easily repair a burst water pipe without having to dig up the main road. The skill of these medieval builders is still admired by visitors to the underground passages today.

▼ An artist's reconstruction of the building of an underground passage at Exeter in the 1490s

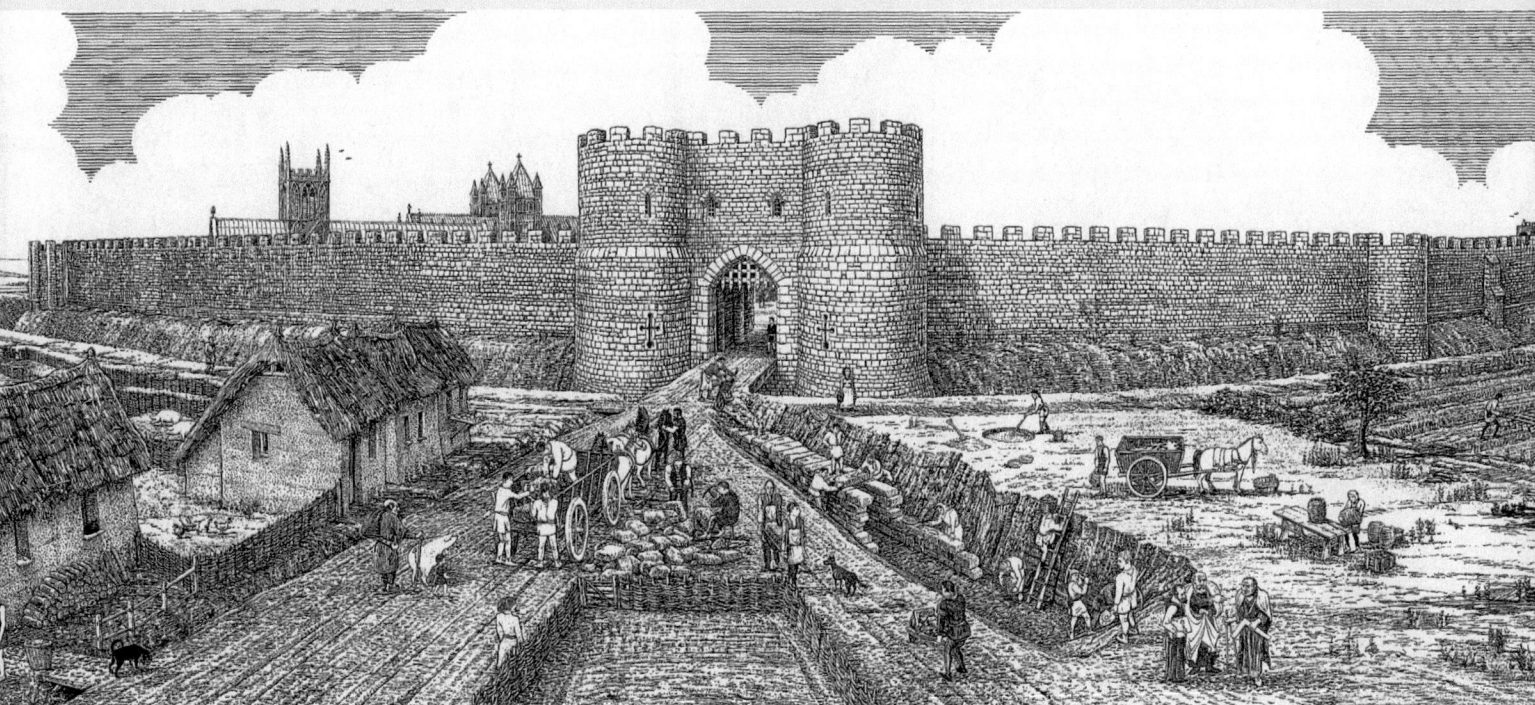

2 The people's health, 1500–1750

More of the same?

The picture below provides a fascinating panorama of London in the early seventeenth century. On the River Thames, watermen in rowing boats take people from one part of the city to another. Sailing ships bring goods to London from different parts of Britain, Europe and the wider world. London Bridge, the only bridge across the river, is packed with houses and shops. If you look carefully, you will find the heads of criminals displayed on pikes above the entrance to the bridge. On the north side of the river you can see St Paul's Cathedral and a host of towers and spires rising from London's many parish churches. On the south bank of the river there are the theatres, alehouses and brothels where Londoners go for their entertainment. There are also two sunken pits where they pay to watch dogs attack bulls and bears.

In the period 1500–1750, London grew into the largest and busiest city in Europe. In 1550, the population of London was around 120,000. By 1650, there were 375,000 people living in the city. London had become a magnificent centre of government, trade, manufacturing, education and entertainment. But, in the year 1665, the people of London suffered a devastating blow: plague returned. There had been many outbreaks of plague in London since the Black Death of 1348, but none was

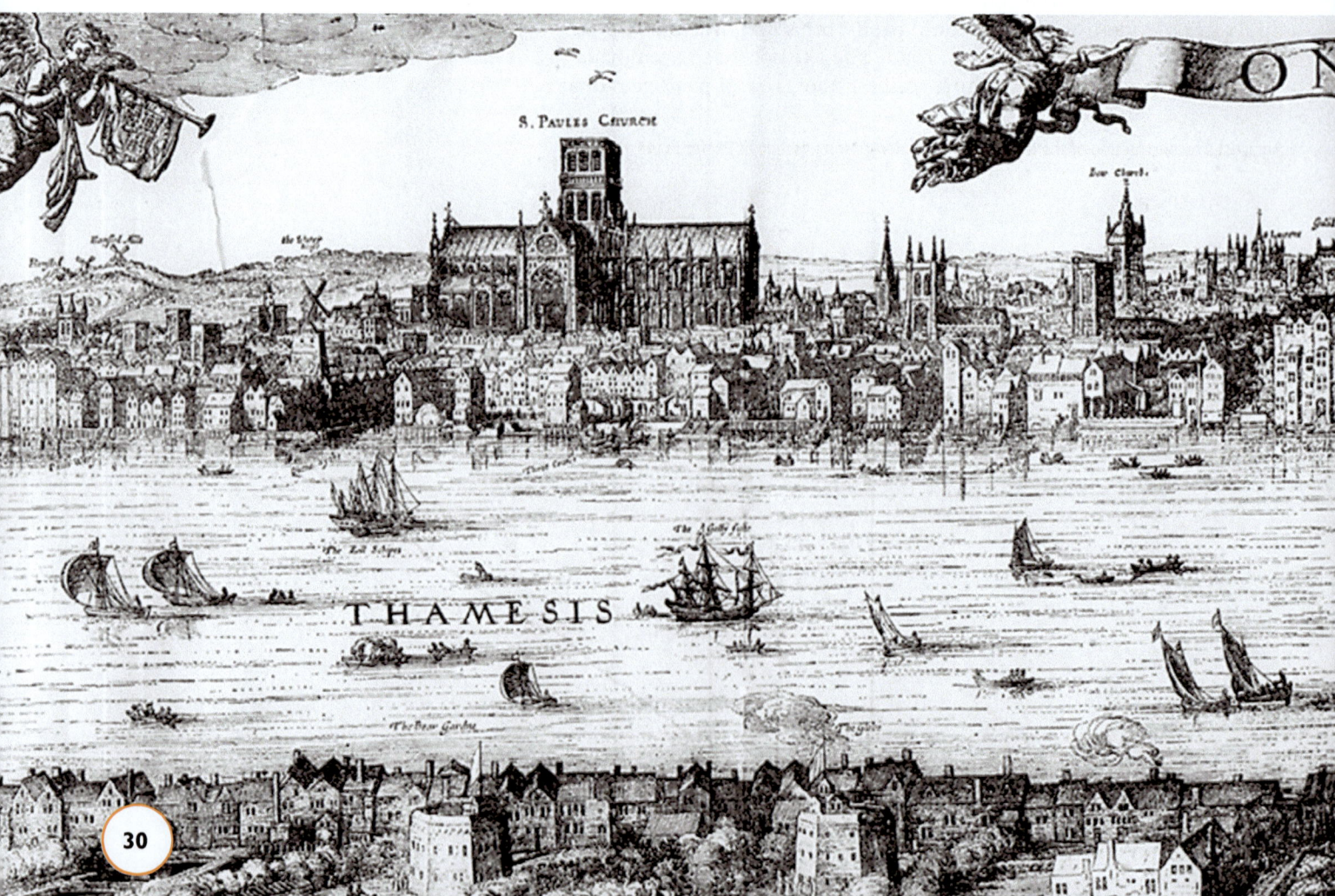

as terrible as the 1665 epidemic. In the spring of that year, people in the poor and crowded parish of St Giles were the first to die of the disease. Through the hot, dry summer of 1665 the plague raged. By September, more than 1,000 people a day were dying. Historians think that between 70,000 and 100,000 Londoners died in the Great Plague of 1665.

The Enquiry

The Great Plague of 1665 which caused so many deaths in London continued to kill people in towns and villages throughout the years 1666 and 1667. After that date, plague never returned to England. This was an important turning point, but it was just one part of the story of people's health in the years between 1500 and 1750. In the early modern period, there were some significant changes in the people's health, but also many continuities. At the end of this enquiry you will have to decide how much had actually changed by 1750. You will focus on three important issues:

1. How changes in people's living conditions in the period 1500–1750 affected their health.
2. Whether people's responses to plague in the period 1500–1750 were very different from their responses in the Middle Ages.
3. How far the authorities in the early modern period made improvements to public health.

But first it will be useful to find out about the bigger changes and continuities in early modern England, and to think about how these might have affected the people's health …

▼ An engraving of London by Claes Visscher, 1616

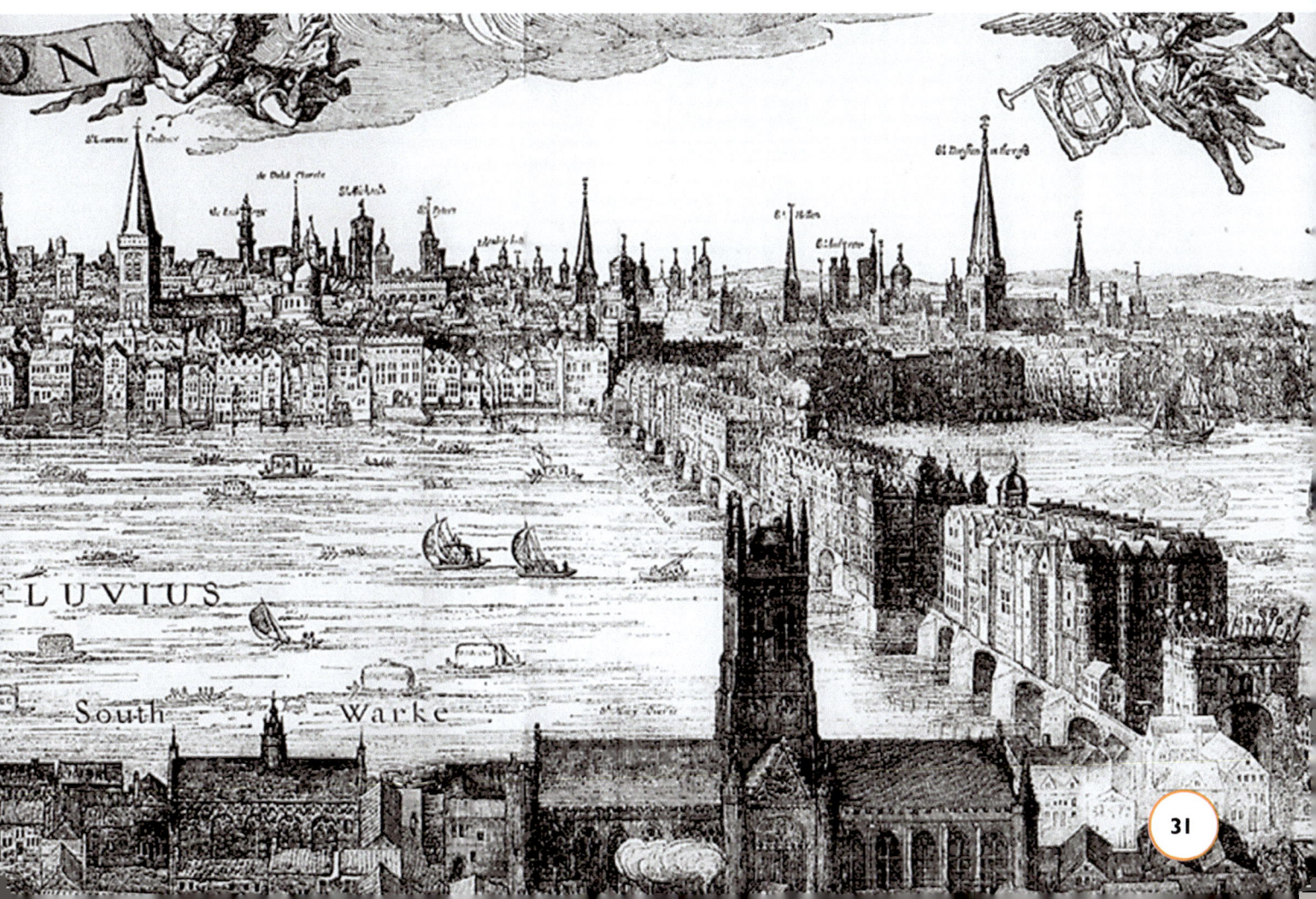

Britain 1500–1750: an overview

Record

The next four pages summarise different aspects of life in Britain, 1500–1750. Read through them quickly and make a list of at least six specific features that you think may have affected people's health at that time. Collect and explain your ideas in a table like this:

Specific feature of life at this time	How I think this may have affected the people's health

1. Daily bread

This detail from an early eighteenth century painting shows men and women harvesting hay at Dixton in Gloucestershire. In the period 1500–1750, most people continued to live and work in the countryside. As you can see, farming was still done by hand and many people were needed to work in the fields at harvest time. If bad weather ruined the harvest there was a shortage of bread and people went hungry. By the eighteenth century, however, hardly anyone died of starvation as they had done in previous centuries. The population of England doubled from around 3 million in 1550 to nearly 6 million in 1750, but improvements in agriculture meant that by the 1700s there was just enough food for this growing population, even in bad years.

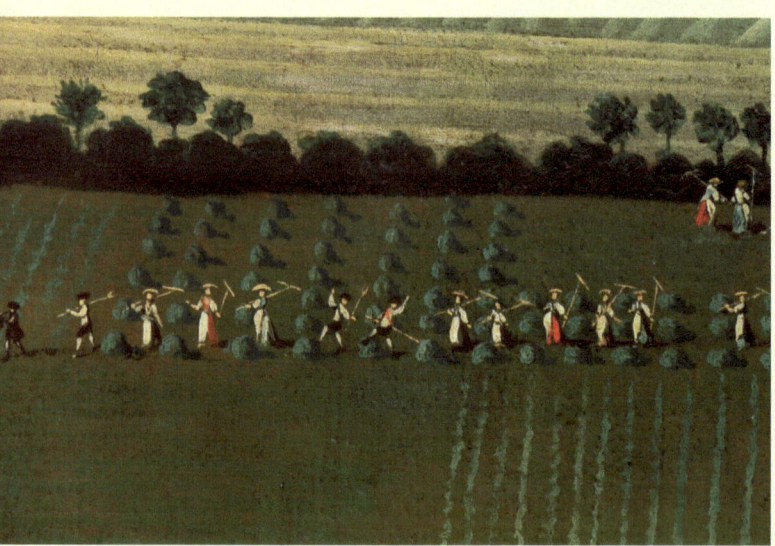

◀ Detail from a painting of harvesters at Dixton, Gloucestershire, early eighteenth century

2. Work

In the early modern period, most people wore woollen clothes, just as they had done in the Middle Ages. This woodcut from the early seventeenth century shows a woman using a spinning wheel to make yarn from wool. The making of woollen cloth was still England's main industry and many people continued to work in their own homes, spinning yarn on wheels and weaving woollen cloth on handlooms. Early modern England was still a pre-industrial country. The age of factories and mass industrialisation would not arrive until 1750–1900.

▶ An early-seventeenth-century woodcut of a woman spinning

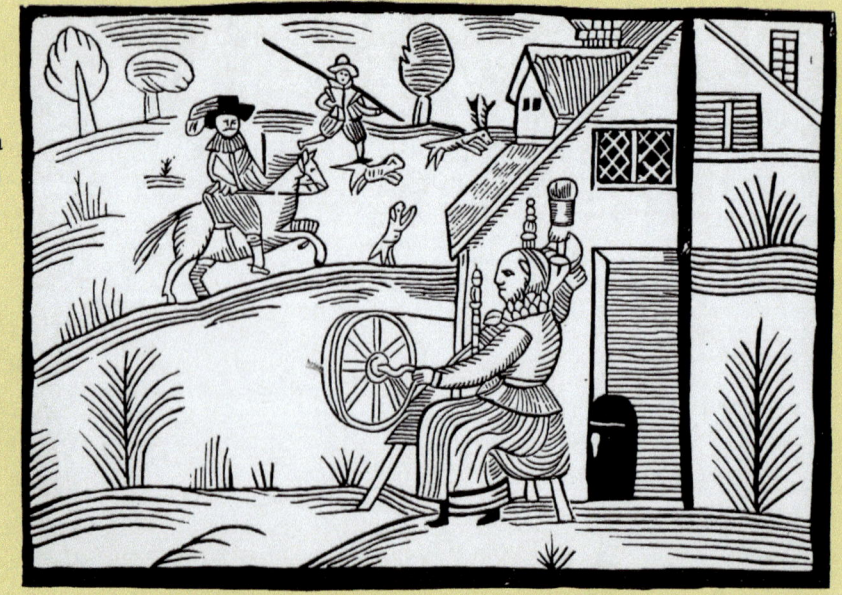

More of the same?

3. Coal

This is a picture of the steam engine which Thomas Newcomen invented in 1712. Hundreds of Newcomen engines were in use by 1750, mainly to pump water out of coal mines. In the seventeenth century, coal was used in the brewing, salt-boiling and glass-making industries, and also as fuel by poor labourers. Coal mines in the north east of England began to produce more coal which was shipped to London and other towns for people to burn on their fires. The problem of air pollution had begun.

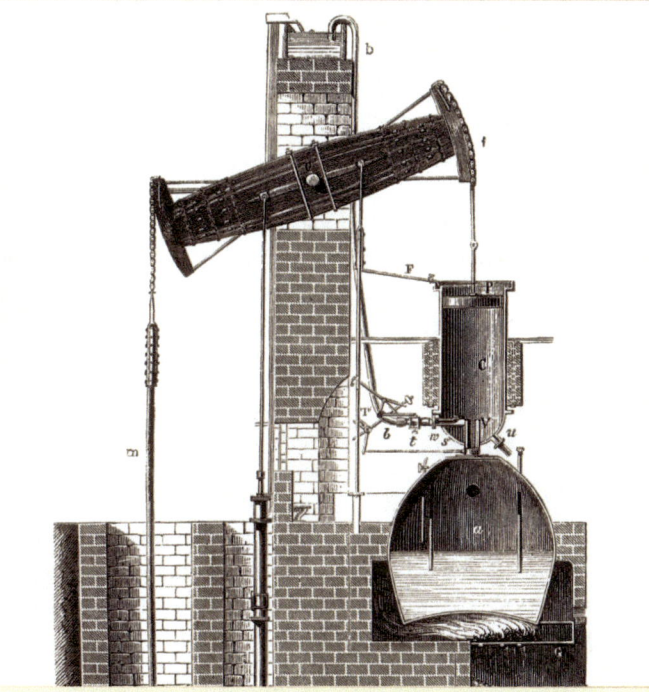

▶ An engraving of Newcomen's steam engine, 1712

4. New products

This painting shows Bristol quay in the eighteenth century. By 1750, Bristol had become an important trading port and the town had more than doubled in size since 1600. The period from 1600 to 1750 saw a transformation in trade with the wider world. In the seventeenth and eighteenth centuries England established colonies in North America and on British plantations in the Caribbean enslaved African people were forced to work to produce goods like sugar and tobacco that the British could trade. In 1608, the East India Company sent its first ship to India and began to exploit its resources to trade in spices, dyes, silk and cotton.

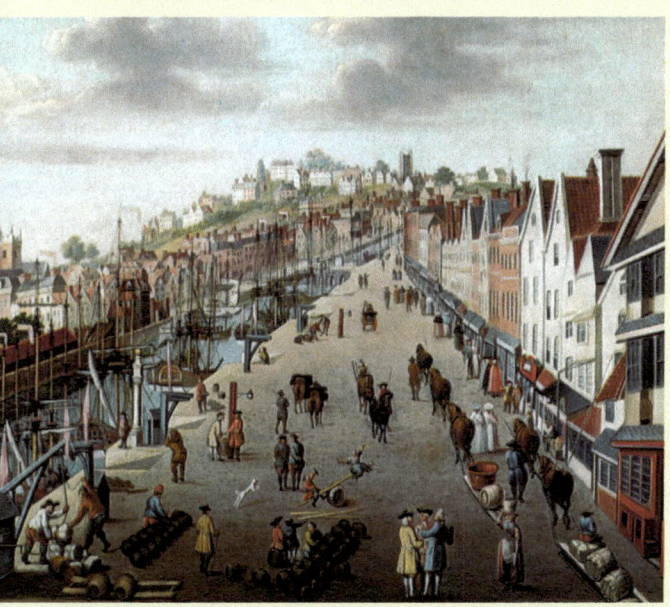

◀ A painting of Bristol Quay in the eighteenth century

5. Growing towns

This map shows the city of Bath in 1694. In 1650 Bath's population of just over 1,000 was tiny. By 1700, the number of people in Bath had doubled and the city had begun to burst out of its old medieval walls. In the early modern period, towns grew quickly as more and more people moved from the countryside to seek work in the urban centres. These people often clustered in overcrowded suburbs outside the city walls. By 1750, about a fifth of the population lived in towns. But remember that this was a relatively minor change compared with the age of mass urbanisation which occurred in the period 1750–1900.

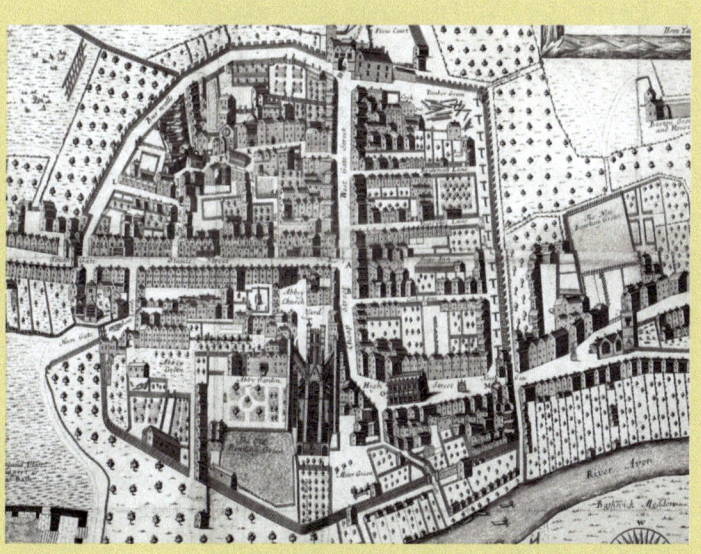

▶ The mathematician Joseph Gilmore's map of Bath, 1694

6. End of the monasteries

These are the ruins of Glastonbury Abbey in Somerset, the largest of over 500 monasteries in England at the end of the Middle Ages. Between 1536 and 1540, Henry VIII and his chief minister, Thomas Cromwell, closed Glastonbury and all the other monasteries in England. They confiscated the treasures of the monasteries and sold their property to local landowners. The monasteries, and their water systems, fell into ruins.

▶ The ruins of Glastonbury Abbey, Somerset

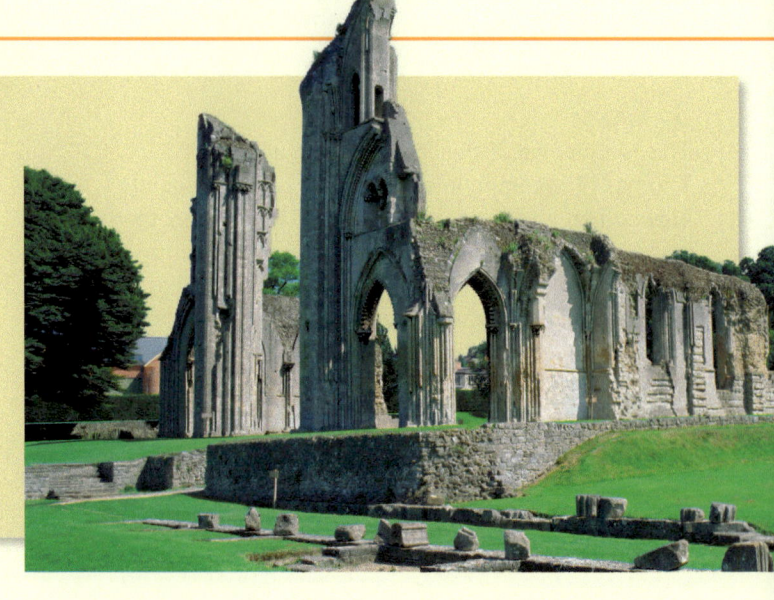

7. New discoveries

People in the early modern period began to search for a scientific way of understanding the world. In the seventeenth century, Robert Hooke developed a powerful microscope and was amazed to discover that plants were made up of small sections which he called 'cells'. In 1665, Hooke's book *Micrographia* was published. It contained a collection of images seen through his microscope, including this picture of a magnified flea. In 1683, a Dutchman called van Leeuwenhoek saw something even more amazing through his own microscope – tiny organisms which we now call germs. This was an important discovery, but it would be another 200 years before a scientist made the connection between germs and disease. In the early modern period scientists still had no understanding of the true cause of plague and other diseases.

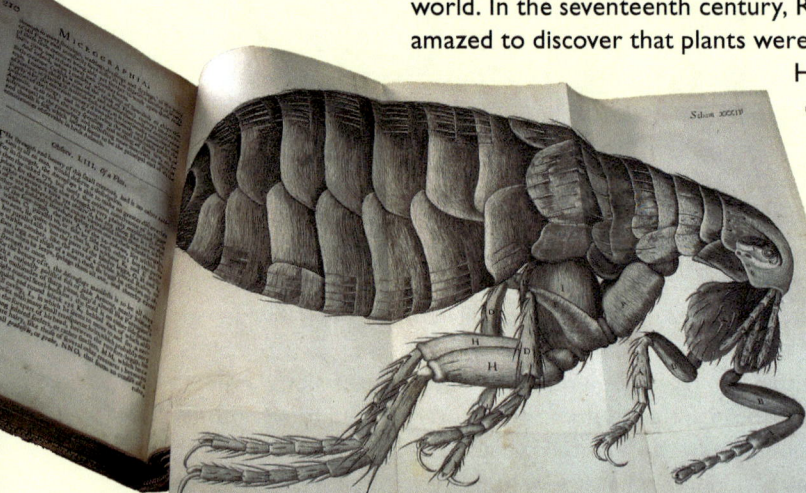

◀ A page from Robert Hooke's *Micrographia*, 1665

8. New printing, but old beliefs

The printing press, which was introduced into England at the end of the fifteenth century, transformed people's lives. For centuries, monks had carefully copied individual manuscripts onto parchment. From the sixteenth century, multiple copies of paper books and pamphlets could be made quickly and cheaply. Printing meant that old thinking could be challenged and new ideas could spread quickly, especially as there were growing numbers of people in early modern England who could read. However, some old ideas were slow to disappear. This picture from a pamphlet printed in 1655 shows the execution of several women who were found guilty of witchcraft. Many people continued to believe in witches during the sixteenth and seventeenth centuries and there was a widely held view that supernatural forces were behind accidents, bad harvests and disease.

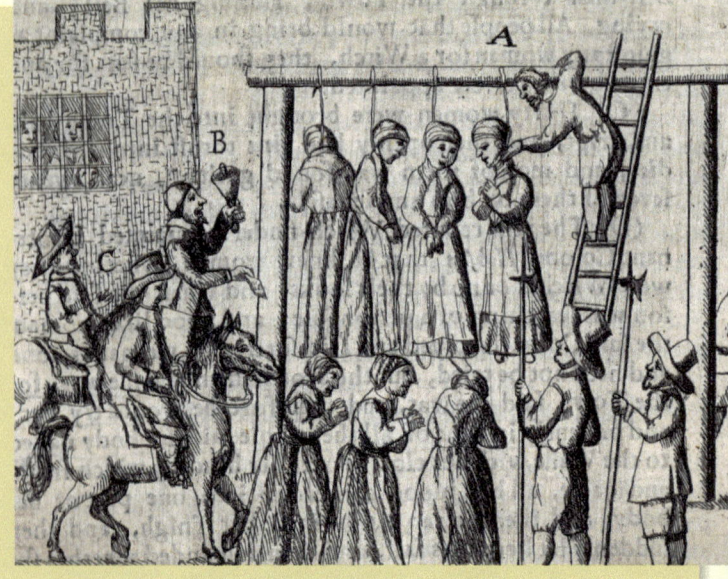

▲ Witches being hanged. From a pamphlet printed in 1655

9. Growing power of parliament

This picture from the late sixteenth century shows Elizabeth I and her parliament. Between 1500 and 1750, monarchs continued to play an important role in government, although parliament was much more powerful than it had been in the Middle Ages. The number of MPs increased, but this made little difference to ordinary people. In the early eighteenth century only 3 per cent of adults could vote in elections. Parliament began to make laws which affected different aspects of people's lives.

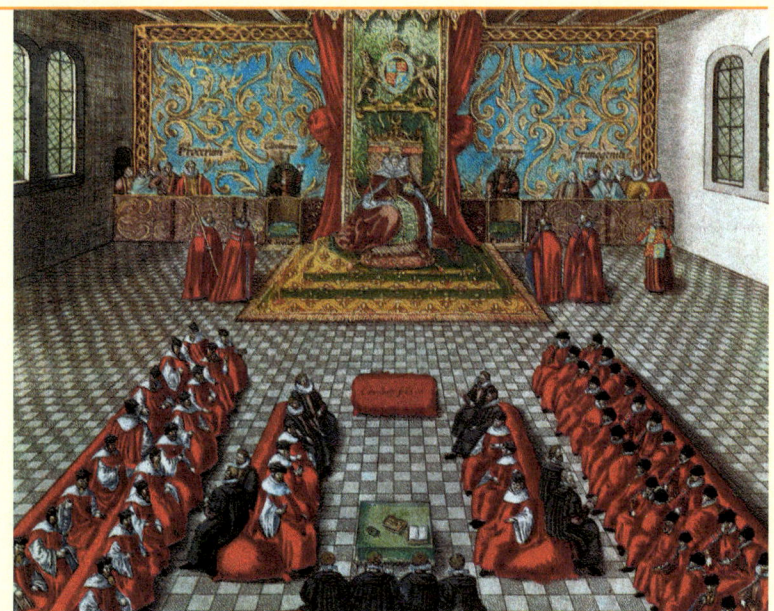

▶ Elizabeth I and her parliament, c.1600

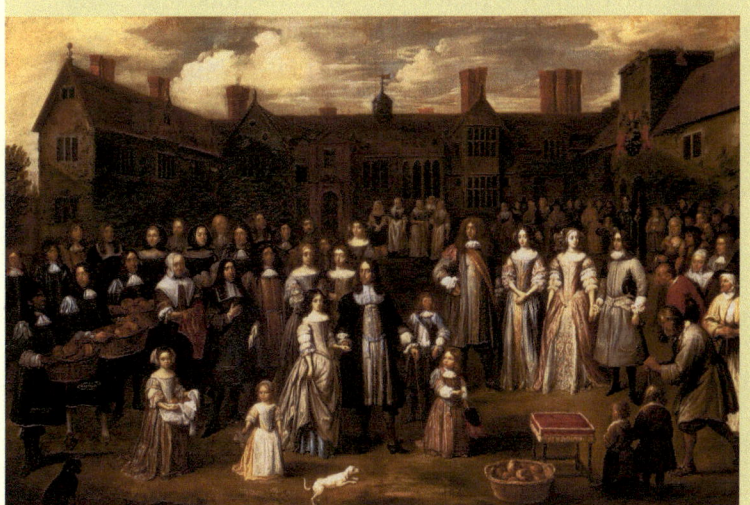

▲ 'The Tichborne Dole', a painting from 1670

10. Power in the localities

This painting from 1670 shows Sir Henry Tichborne handing out bread to the poor people on his manor in Hampshire. Large landowners like Sir Henry Tichborne played an important part in running their county, just as they had done in the Middle Ages. In each county, men from landowning families became Justices of the Peace, enforcing the law and acting as administrators. This was an important continuity, but in the early modern period new elite groups such as merchants, lawyers and doctors emerged whose wealth did not depend on land. In towns, it was wealthy merchants who controlled the councils through their roles as mayors and aldermen. When plague struck, these men were expected to take action in their locality.

11. The alehouse

This is Mother Louse, an Oxfordshire alehouse-keeper from the 1650s. You can see her shabby alehouse in the background. The 'common people' of early modern England included a wide range of occupations: yeoman (richer farmers), husbandmen (poorer farmers), tradesmen, craftsmen and poor labourers. These people, like the peasants and craftsmen of medieval times, drank a lot of ale and beer. In the period 1500–1750, the number of alehouses in villages and towns grew rapidly and they became important meeting places. The common people went to the alehouse to eat, dance, gamble, flirt and drink – often to excess. From the 1570s, they could also enjoy a pipe of tobacco, unaware of what it was doing to their lungs.

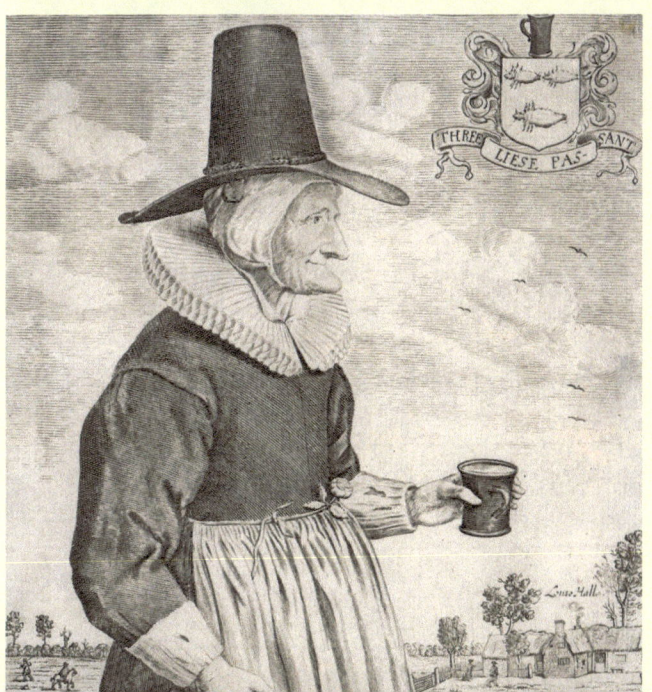

◀ 'Mother Louse', an engraving from the 1650s

How did living conditions in the period 1500–1750 affect people's health?

Record

To help you think about this question, read the information on the next six pages and make bullet point notes under the following headings:

Food and famine	The urban environment	Clean water	Waste

Include main points and examples. Remember to include comments on how different aspects of people's living conditions affected their health.

Food and famine

In 1567, Lord Cobham commissioned this portrait of himself and his family. He used the portrait to show off the expensive clothes, exotic pets and fine foods he could afford for himself and his family. Elizabeth, his five-year-old daughter, is about to eat a bowl of cherries. Frances, her twin, is tucking into an apple. On the table in front of the girls is a plate of pears, apples and grapes. Not everyone at that time agreed that eating fresh fruit was a good thing. Some people pointed out that fruit made you fart a lot so it could not be good for you. Others even argued that eating fruit caused plague. In the sixteenth century, just as today, there was conflicting advice about food.

▼ A portrait of Lord Cobham, and his family, 1567

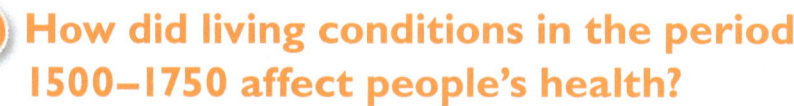

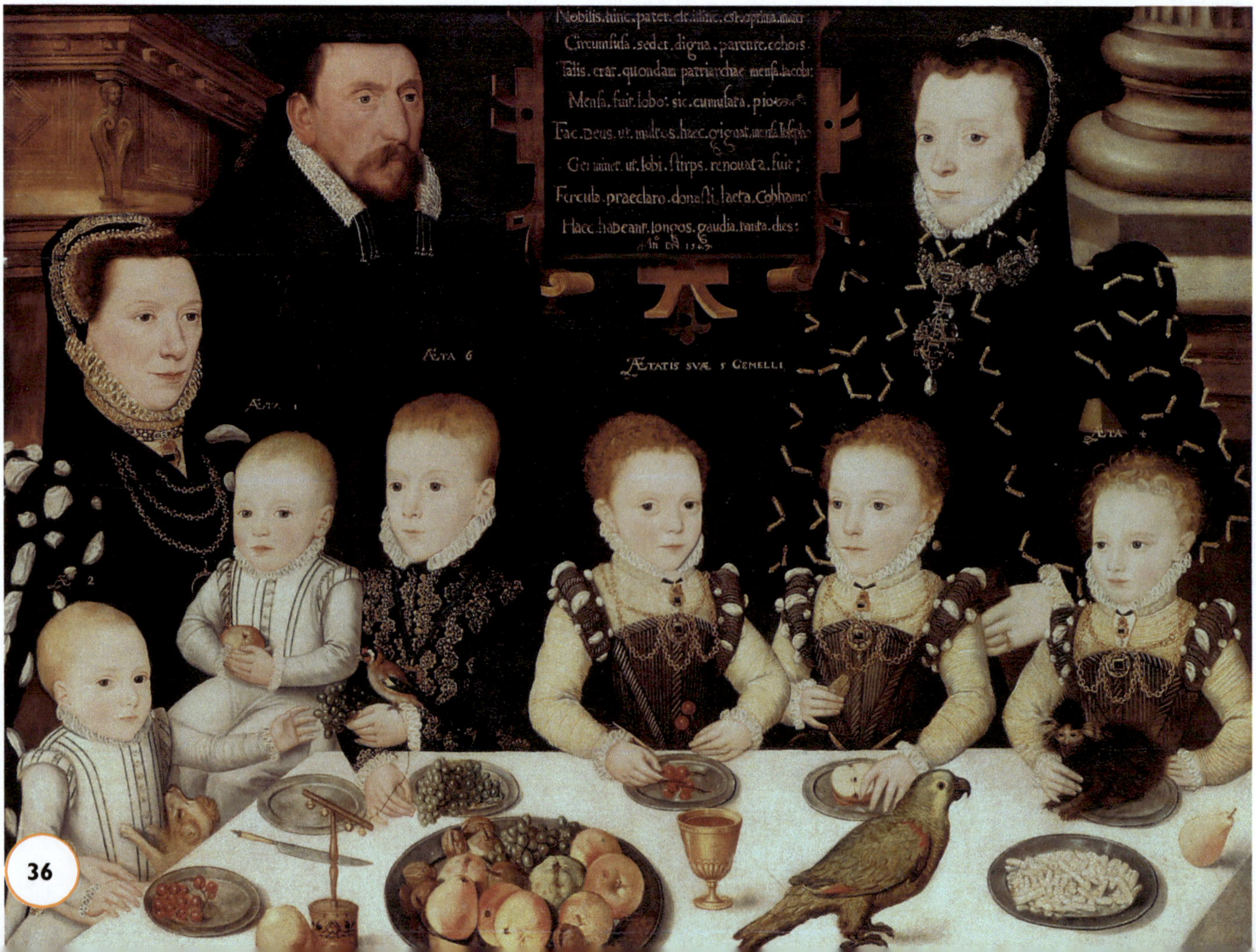

In many ways, the food people enjoyed in the early modern period had not changed much since the Middle Ages. Those who could afford it ate a large quantity, and a wide variety, of meat: beef, veal, mutton, lamb, pork, chicken, goose, rabbit, pigeon and a range of small birds. Fish was an important part of the diet too as the religious custom of eating fish on Friday continued, even after the Reformation. The wealthy enjoyed white bread (which was more like our brown bread nowadays) and their diet included only small quantities of salad leaves, vegetables and fruit. People drank wine, ale, beer or mead as they knew that the water could make them ill. Overall, wealthy people in early modern England had plenty to eat, but their unbalanced diet would give a modern dietician nightmares.

In the early modern period, merchants brought new products to England from America and Asia, and people who could afford it began to eat a wider range of foods. Peppers, pumpkins, chillies, tomatoes and potatoes all appeared on the tables of the wealthy. New drinks like hot chocolate, tea and coffee became popular, all sweetened with sugar produced by enslaved African people on British plantations in the Caribbean. By 1750 there were over 500 coffee houses in London. The national addiction to coffee and sugar had well and truly begun. So too had the problems of rotting teeth and obesity.

The diet of poorer people was mainly bread and vegetables with eggs, cheese, fish or meat as occasional treats. Pottage (a thick vegetable soup) was widely eaten by the labouring poor, just as it had been by medieval peasants. Throughout the early modern period, a labourer's daily wage was barely enough to feed his family. When bad weather ruined the harvest, the price of grain rocketed and labouring families struggled to buy bread. If there was a run of bad harvests, people could starve to death. You can see evidence of this in the 1623 register of burials from the village of Greystoke, Cumbria. Widespread famine like the one which occurred in 1623–24 was rare in early modern England, but hunger which weakened people's resistance to disease was common.

> **Reflect**
> What interesting details can you find in this extract from the parish register of Greystoke?

Selected burials in the parish register of Greystoke, Cumbria, 1623

27 March: A poor hungerstarved beggar child, Dorothy, daughter of Henry Patterson, miller.

28 March: Thomas Simpson, a poor, hungerstarved beggar boy and son of one Richard Simpson of Brough.

12 July: Thomas, child of Richard Bell, a poor man, which child died for very want of food and maintenance to live.

27 September: John, son of John Lancaster, late of Greystoke, a waller by trade, which child died for want of food and means.

4 October: Agnes, wife of John Lancaster, late of Greystoke, a waller by trade, which woman died for want of means to live.

> **Record**
> Use the information on food and famine to start your bullet point notes. Your first main point could be:
>
> Wealthy people had a varied diet

The urban environment

In the early modern period, people in towns bought their food from shops, markets and street sellers. In an age before freezers and plastic packaging, food did not stay fresh for very long, and the chances of food poisoning were high. In this c.1984 painting, the artist Ivan Lapper depicted a sixteenth-century street market. The artist's interpretation also included other interesting features of the urban environment.

Record

Use the information on the urban environment to make your notes. Your first point could be:

> People often bought their food from street sellers.

Animals

During the hours of daylight, the main streets of towns were always crowded as people from different social groups mingled and went about their business. In early modern towns a bear might have been unusual, but people shared the streets with animals. Cattle, sheep and geese were herded through the streets to be sold or slaughtered. Horse-drawn carts blocked the way and sometimes injured or killed small children. The many loose dogs were a particular problem as their excrement contains parasites that could be spread to humans. Cats were common, but they could not control the rats and mice which flourished in early modern towns.

Streets

This picture is so crowded with people and animals that it is hard to see the street surface. Often streets were just beaten earth or gravel, which turned to dust in summer and to mud as soon as it rained. Main streets like the one in the picture were sometimes paved with stone or cobbled, but paved streets were often covered in animal dung. Before the eighteenth century, there were very few raised pavements so people's clothes and shoes were often very dirty after walking in the street.

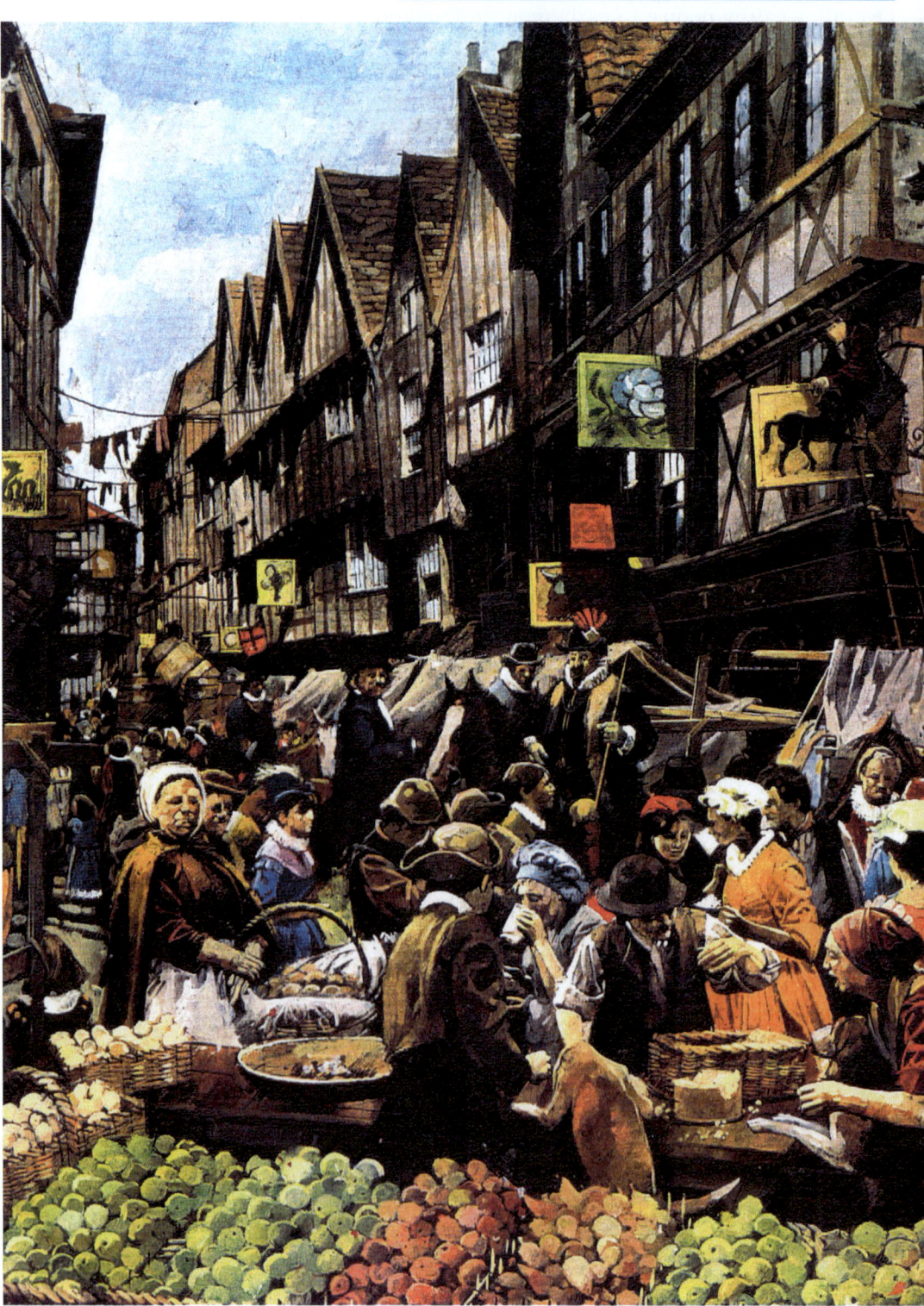

▶ A painting of a sixteenth-century street, by the artist Ivan Lapper, c.1984

More of the same?

Smoke
Perhaps because the artist has chosen to set the picture in summer, one thing missing from the picture is smoke. If you look carefully you will find chimney-sweeps at work. In the period 1500–1750, people heated their houses and did their cooking on open fires. In the sixteenth century, coal was unpopular because it gave off a foul smell when burnt, but when the price of coal dropped in the seventeenth century more people began to burn it on their fires. Urban craftsmen also burnt coal in their ovens, forges and furnaces. The dust, soot and smoke from chimneys in early modern towns contributed to respiratory diseases.

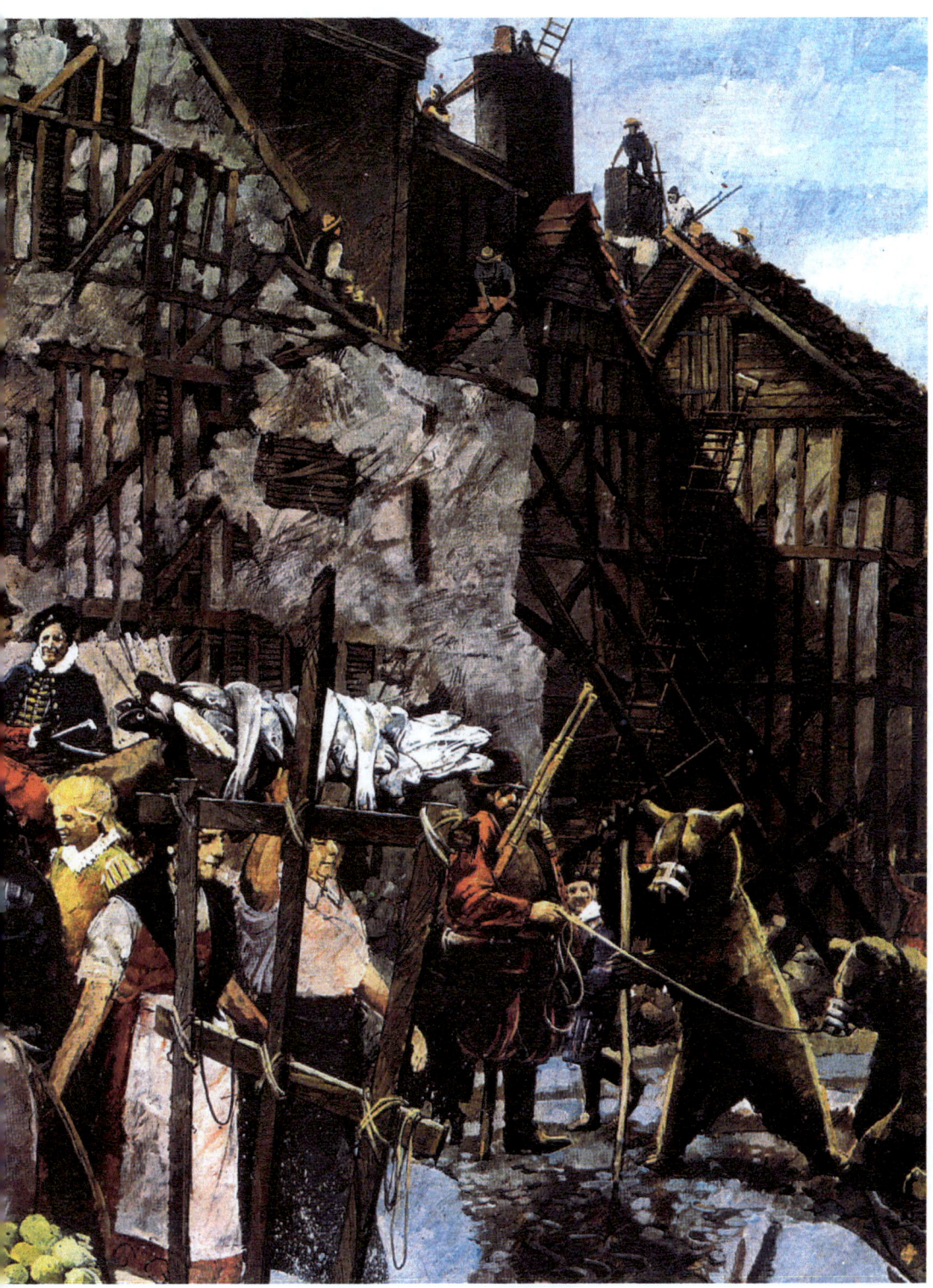

Houses
In the sixteenth century, the inhabitants of many towns continued to live in medieval oak-framed houses like the ones in the picture. From the seventeenth century, these were gradually replaced by houses built from stone or brick. Houses in towns were often just one room wide and three storeys tall. Some had overhanging 'jetties' on the top storey to provide more space. Many houses were overcrowded. Poor families squashed into cellars and upper storeys, and sharing beds was common. Houses continued to be poorly constructed in the early modern period and this meant that they were often draughty and damp. No wonder many people suffered from respiratory diseases.

Clean water

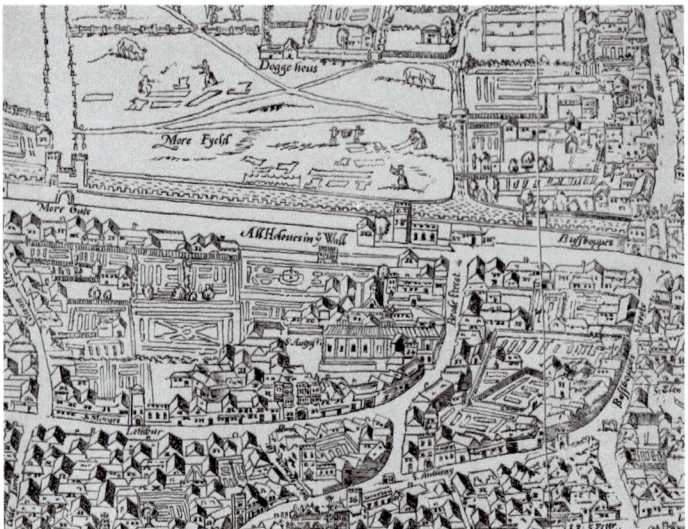

▲ Detail from a sixteenth-century map of London. Probably made by Ralph Agas in the 1560s

> **Reflect**
>
> This is a detail from the oldest surviving map of London, probably made by Ralph Agas in the 1560s. Look carefully and find the women drying washing on Moor Field. Why do you think washing was dried this way?

The inclusion of women drying washing in Ralph Agas's map suggests that people in sixteenth-century London cared about keeping their clothes and sheets clean. But cleanliness in the early modern period depended on your wealth. Richer people and the 'middling sort' had servants to do their washing. A poor labourer might only have one set of woollen clothes. When dirty, his clothes would be riddled with lice and fleas – the carriers of typhus and plague.

It is difficult to know exactly how people in early modern England kept their bodies clean, but it seems that our modern habit of having a shower or bath at the beginning of the day was not part of people's daily routine in the period 1500–1750. There were three reasons for this:

1. If you lived near a river or pond you could always take a quick cold dip, but bathing inside was only possible if you had a bathtub, servants, a reliable water supply, enough firewood and plenty of time.
2. Soap made from the leftover animal fat of candle makers could be used for washing clothes, but it was not suitable for use on the skin. Only the rich could afford soap made from olive oil.
3. The water would often be dirty and many people believed that water could infect them through the pores in their skin.

For these reasons, cleaning the body was often a dry process, using a brush or linen cloth to rub the skin and dislodge any lice.

In the countryside, people could carry clean water from wells, springs or streams. As towns expanded, obtaining clean water became a problem. Some people were lucky enough to have a well in their garden or yard. Otherwise there were three main ways to get access to water:

1. **Paying for water to be piped to your house**. In some towns, companies constructed pipes made from elm or lead in order to bring water from distant springs. In 1609, for example, Hugh Middleton built a 'New River' which brought spring water 38 miles from the countryside outside London to a reservoir in Islington from which 30,000 houses in the city could be supplied. People paid a quarterly bill to be connected to the pipes.

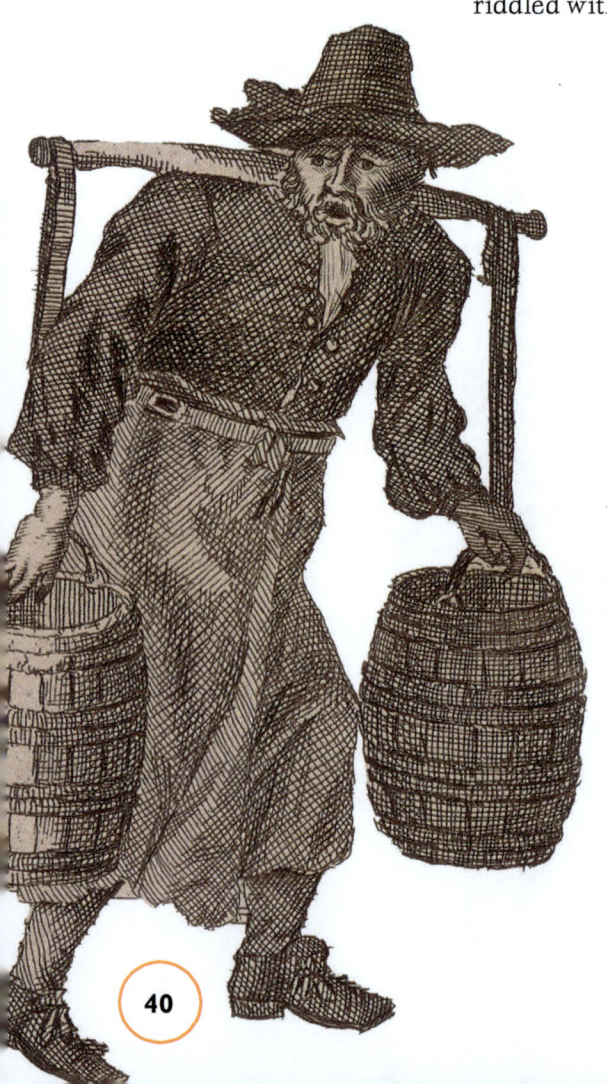

▼ A seventeenth-century illustration of a London water-seller

2. **Collecting water from a conduit.** Conduits were public water fountains provided by town councils or by individuals as acts of charity. There were smaller versions of conduits known as 'bosses' which were sometimes built into walls. People helped themselves to the water free of charge.
3. **Buying water from a water-seller.** Water-sellers collected water from conduits or the river and carried it through the streets in a large container like the one in the picture opposite. You could pay a water-seller to bring water to your house.

However people obtained their water in early modern towns, it must have tasted terrible and would have been unsafe to drink. No wonder people preferred to drink small (weak) beer.

> **Record**
>
> Use the information on **water** to add to your notes (see page 36). Your first main point could be:
>
> Wealthy people had servants to wash their clothes.

Waste

People in early modern England produced a lot less rubbish than we do with all our modern packaging. Town-dwellers could put household waste – food, paper, sweepings, dirty rushes from the floor and ash from the fire – outside their house in a basket or tub. Once or twice a week, it was collected by 'scavengers' (sometimes called 'rakers') who sold urban waste to market gardeners outside the towns. If you forgot to put out your waste you could always tip it on one of the common dunghills that were found outside the gates of early modern towns.

Getting rid of urine and excrement (commonly known as piss and shit in the early modern period) was a difficult business. In 1596, Sir John Harrington, Queen Elizabeth I's godson, invented the first flushing water closet (toilet), but people needed their own drains and a plentiful supply of water in order to install one. Water closets were not widely used in the early modern period, although some wealthier people began to have them fitted in the eighteenth century.

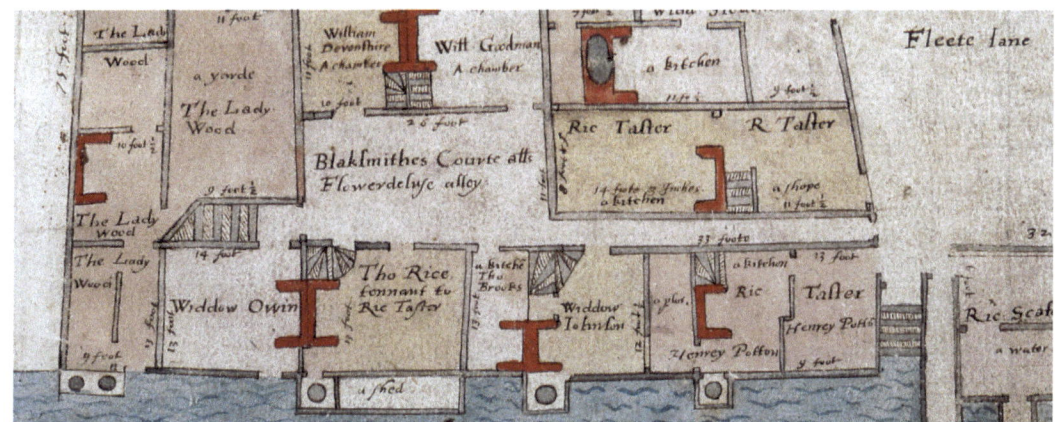

◀ Detail from Ralph Treswell's survey, 1612

Nearly everyone in early modern England continued to use privies as their ancestors had done in the Middle Ages. In the countryside little changed, but in the growing towns getting rid of excrement became an increasing problem. If your house backed onto a river or ditch you might have considered building a privy (sometimes called a 'jakes') over the water. Five of the many jakes built over London's Fleet Ditch are shown on the plan above, made in 1612. Most people, however, used a privy built over a cesspit in their garden, yard or sometimes inside the house. Cesspits sometimes leaked, causing problems for neighbours. On the morning of 20 October 1660, Samuel Pepys stepped into 'a great heap of turds' which had leaked into his cellar from a neighbour's cesspit.

Every year or two a cesspit would need to be emptied. This unpleasant task was done by the scavengers, usually at night. Emptying a cesspit was an expensive job which often required barrels of excrement to be carried through the house. Poorer people sometimes emptied their own cesspits, creating dunghills in back yards and alleys.

> **Record**
>
> Use the information on **waste** to complete your notes. Your first main point could be:
>
> In towns people could put their rubbish on the street for the 'scavengers' to collect.'

Responses to plague

In sixteenth-century England, the average life expectancy was only 41 years. Of course, many people lived to be much older than this. It was the huge number of infant and child deaths which led to such a low average life expectancy. A number of killer diseases caused high mortality in early modern England.

> **Reflect**
>
> Which of the diseases below were linked to people's living conditions?

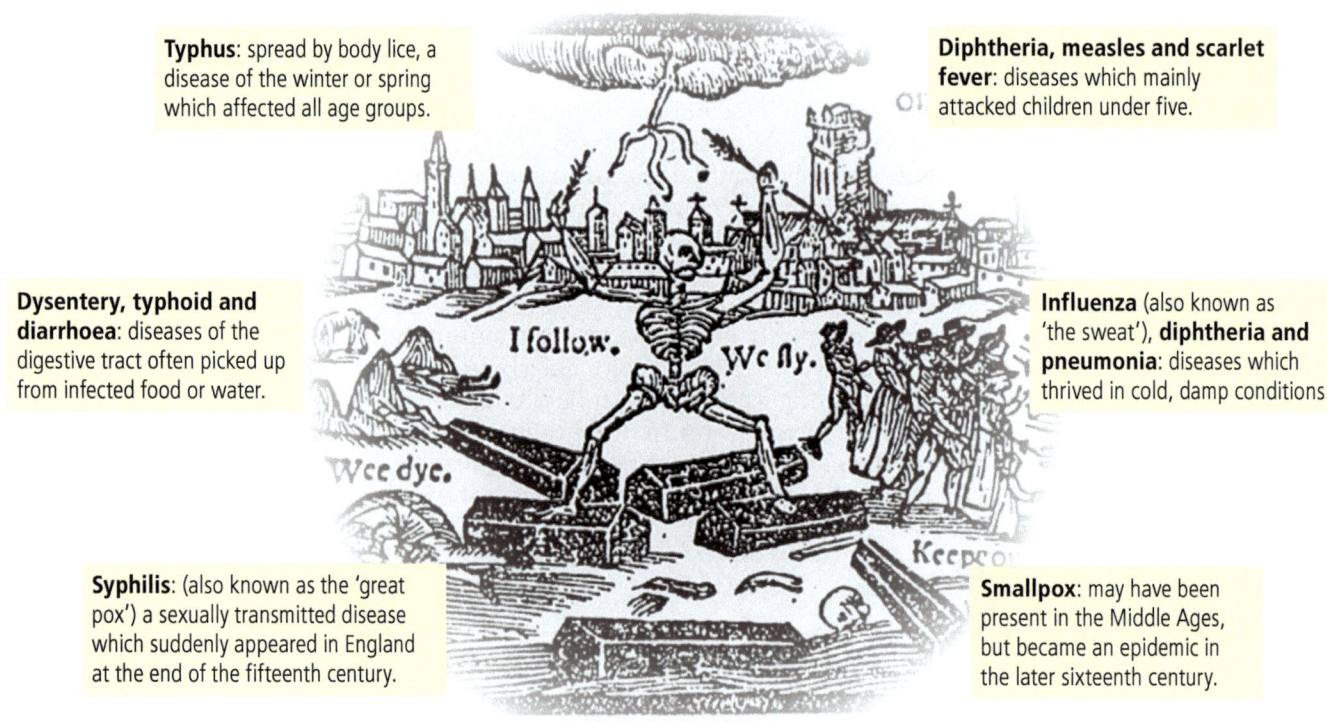

Typhus: spread by body lice, a disease of the winter or spring which affected all age groups.

Diphtheria, measles and scarlet fever: diseases which mainly attacked children under five.

Dysentery, typhoid and diarrhoea: diseases of the digestive tract often picked up from infected food or water.

Influenza (also known as 'the sweat'), **diphtheria and pneumonia**: diseases which thrived in cold, damp conditions.

Syphilis: (also known as the 'great pox') a sexually transmitted disease which suddenly appeared in England at the end of the fifteenth century.

Smallpox: may have been present in the Middle Ages, but became an epidemic in the later sixteenth century.

These diseases were awful but by far the most terrifying disease in the early modern period was still the plague.

- **Plague was terrifying because of its *frequency*.**

Plague in England began with the Black Death of 1348–49 and neared its end with the so-called 'Great Plague' of 1665. In the early modern period, plague was not as severe as it had been in the Middle Ages, but it never went away. One historian has calculated that there were at least eight major outbreaks of plague in the years between 1500 and 1670 – in other words, one outbreak every twenty years. There were particularly widespread epidemics in the 1540s and 1550s, the late 1590s and in the first decade of the seventeenth century. In the early modern period, plague could still strike villages, but it increasingly became a disease of towns where rats were most common. Bristol, for example, experienced serious epidemics in 1597, 1603, 1637–38, 1643, 1650–51 and 1666. Early modern people knew that there was always the possibility of a plague epidemic and must have dreaded a new outbreak of the disease.

- **Plague was terrifying because of its symptoms.**

Once again, it was the bubonic plague that was most common. Its effects on the human body were well known. The first sign of the disease was a blister appearing where the victim had been bitten by a flea. This soon became a gangrenous, blackish carbuncle. The victim's temperature rose to around 40°C and this was followed by headaches, vomiting, great thirst and terrible pain. At the same time, more signs of the disease appeared on the skin. The lymph nodes, usually in the groin but sometimes in the armpit and neck, swelled with pus and formed large buboes. More carbuncles appeared on different parts of the body along with blisters and large red, blue, purple and black blotches under the skin. The heart and kidneys began to fail and the victim became delirious. Only one in five people who caught the plague survived. After the first flea bite, death usually came in five days.

- **Plague was terrifying because of its impact.**

Plague struck suddenly. It mostly began in spring with the arrival of warmer weather. In the summer months, when rats and fleas flourished, the number of deaths increased rapidly. The disease often killed ten per cent of people in a community in less than a year. In the worst cases, the death rate could be a third or more of the population. The poorest neighbourhoods or towns were the worst affected and the impact on individual families in these areas could be catastrophic. The 1665 plague in Cambridge had a devastating effect on one poor family in the riverside and rat-infested parish of St Clements. On 1 September, the teenager Daniel Pawston was the first of his family to die of the plague. The Pawston house was nailed shut with the words 'Lord Have Mercy on Us' painted across the door. Inside were Daniel's parents, his brothers Samuel and Luke and their big sister Alice, aged 15. By 18 September, all four Pawston children and their parents had died of the plague.

- **Plague was terrifying because nobody understood it.**

Early modern people tried to understand what caused plague so that they could fight against it. The number of printed medical books and pamphlets increased hugely after 1550, but medical knowledge about the cause of the disease made little progress. People continued to believe that God sent the plague as a punishment for people's sins. They thought that God created particular star formations which caused foul air known as 'miasma'. Miasma could also be caused by unburied corpses, stagnant water or the filthy streets. Dirty clothes or the fur of dogs and cats could spread miasma from one place to another. At the end of the seventeenth century, some writers began to emphasise the importance of contagion (close contact with an infected person) as a way of spreading the disease, but they also clung on to the theory of miasma. These natural and supernatural explanations for disease had serious limitations. Most importantly, **there was still no understanding of the role of rats and fleas in spreading the plague**.

After 1667, plague never returned to England. No-one is quite sure why this happened. Perhaps the most likely explanation is that effective measures in Europe to stop the spread of plague meant that the disease no longer spread to England. Whatever the reason, people in England were free from plague for the first time in over 400 years. They, of course, did not know it.

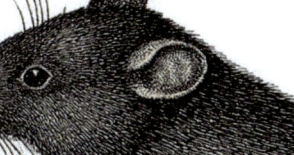

▼ A black rat

Record

Draw a simple cartoon of the face of someone from the seventeenth century who looks terrified by the threat of plague. Surround the face with thought bubbles showing why the person was terrified.

How national government responded to the plague

> **Record**
>
> Use what you learn on the next two pages to write a clear and organised summary of the ways in which national and local government responded to plague in early modern England.
>
> Add a final paragraph to explain how far this differed from the Middle Ages.

By 1500, rulers in Scotland, France and the Italian city states had taken measures to prevent the spread of plague. In comparison, England was a backward country with no national precautions in place. However, during the sixteenth and seventeenth centuries, the English government began to learn from its neighbours. The government introduced important measures in 1518, 1578 and 1604 which forced Justices of the Peace and town corporations to take action at times of plague.

In 1518 ...

Henry VIII issued a proclamation which adopted one of the measures used in Europe: isolation. This would become the most important aspect of plague prevention in England for the next 150 years. The proclamation stated that houses infected with plague in London should be clearly identified. Bundles of straw should be hung from the windows of infected houses for a period of forty days. If anyone left the house they had to carry a white stick so that people knew to avoid them in the streets.

The royal proclamation of 1518 was the beginning of a national policy on public health in England. From 1518, mayors and aldermen in all of England's towns were expected to take action when plague struck. As well as shutting up houses where someone had plague, some corporations started to isolate plague victims in 'pesthouses' outside the town walls. During the 1550s, the aldermen in York introduced additional measures. They posted 'watchmen' on the Ouse Bridge to stop the movement of infected people across the town, appointed 'searchers' to bury the dead and clean infected houses, and collected money from each parish in the city to provide food for people in infected houses.

In 1578 ...

The Privy Council of Elizabeth I ordered the printing of Plague Orders which were sent to the counties and towns across England. From the second half of the sixteenth century, the printing press became an important weapon in the government's battle to improve public health. The Plague Orders of 1578 contained seventeen orders which Justices of the Peace and aldermen had to enforce at times of plague. Local authorities printed summaries of the Plague Orders and stuck them on doors and posts for people to read.

Some of the 1578 Plague Orders were:

- Justices and aldermen should meet once every three weeks during epidemics.
- They should appoint 'viewers' or 'searchers' of the dead in each parish who would report on how the infection developed.
- The aldermen should collect money to support the sick in their town.
- Special prayers should be said in church.
- Streets and alleys should be thoroughly cleaned.
- Barrels of tar should be burned in the streets.
- No dogs, cats or tame pigeons should be allowed on the streets.
- The clothes and bedding of plague victims should be burned.
- Funerals should take place at dusk to reduce the number of people attending.
- Infected houses in towns should be completely shut up for at least six weeks, with all members of the family, sick or healthy, still inside. Watchmen should be appointed to enforce this order.

> **Reflect**
>
> What different beliefs lay behind these orders?

The last order in the list above – locking up whole families in infected houses – was a particularly strict policy which caused much controversy at the time. Many people felt that locking up healthy people with the sick was not a good idea. However, this strict policy of locking up whole families in their houses remained in place throughout the period 1578–1667.

In 1604 ...

Parliament passed a law to enforce new plague orders. The Plague Act of 1604 extended the help which was provided to sick families. It allowed towns to collect money first from parishes within a radius of five miles from the town, and then from the whole county if necessary. It also introduced harsh punishments for anyone breaking the policy of isolation. A plague victim found out of their house and mingling with other people could be hanged. A healthy person who left an infected house which had been shut up could be whipped.

More of the same?

Local responses: some evidence

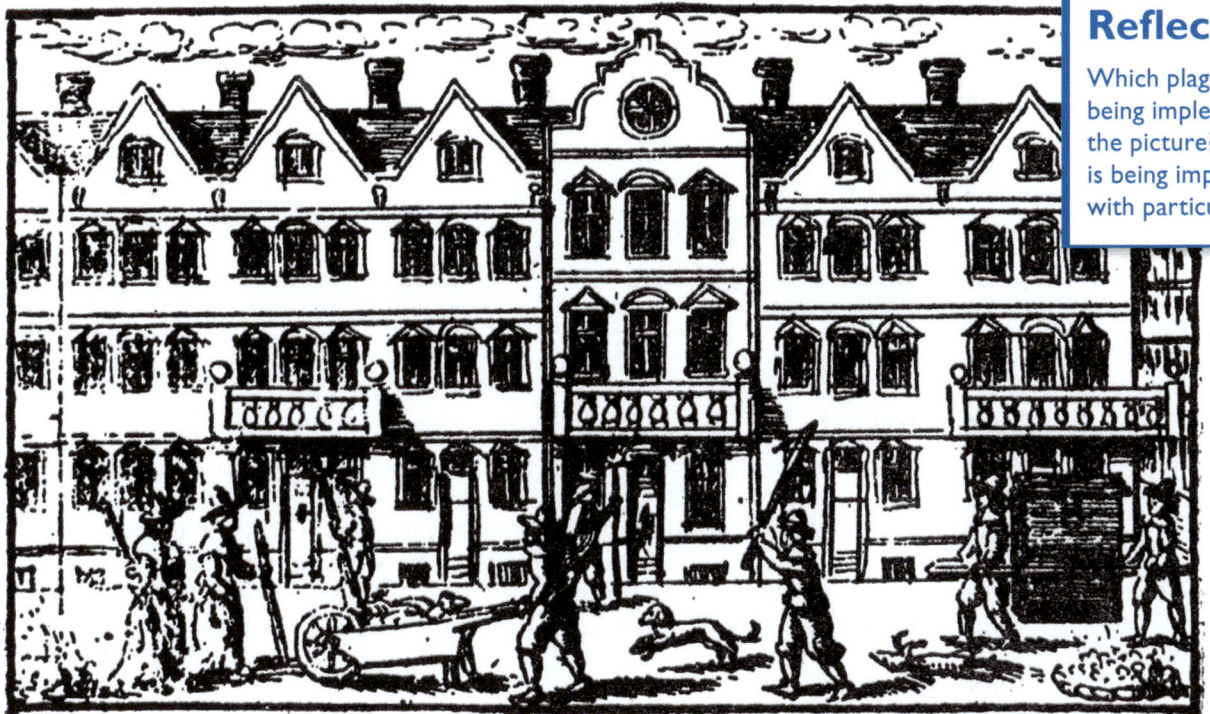

> **Reflect**
> Which plague orders are being implemented in the picture? Which one is being implemented with particular severity?

◀ A seventeenth-century print of a London street during the plague

The first reaction of many town corporations to an outbreak of plague was to pretend it was not happening. However, by the seventeenth century, the policy of isolating the sick and supporting them with food and drink was implemented by most towns in England. More and more towns built pesthouses for plague victims and took a wide range of measures to stop the spread of disease. Cambridge provides a good example. In the spring of 1665, travellers and carriers to Cambridge brought news of the plague which was raging in London. The Cambridge aldermen were prepared. Strangers were only allowed into the town with a certificate of health. The streets were cleaned. Stray dogs and cats were killed. Searchers were hired. The plague's first victim in Cambridge was John Morley who died in one of the town's pesthouses on 25 July 1665. By December 1666 there were 920 bodies in Cambridge's churchyards and pesthouse plague pits.

> **Reflect**
> This is from a 'Bill of Mortality' produced by the authorities in Cambridge during the 1665–66 plague.
> 1. Read the document carefully and work out what a Bill of Mortality was.
> 2. What does it tell us about the response of the authorities in Cambridge to the plague?

▲ From the Cambridge Bills of Mortality, 31 July to 7 August, 1666

The people's reactions

At a time of plague people faced great insecurity. The streets, markets and alehouses emptied. More and more houses were shut up. Day after day, the church bells tolled, reminding people to pray for the souls of neighbours, friends and family who had died.

> **Record**
>
> As you read about these people's behaviour make two lists under these headings:
>
> | 1. Changes from the Middle Ages | 2. Continuities from the Middle Ages |
> | --- | --- |
> | | |

Turning to God

As we might expect, church attendance increased when plague threatened. By the late sixteenth century, England was a Protestant country and people no longer accepted the medieval Catholic responses to disease. English Protestants did not approve of walking barefoot, wearing a hair shirt or going on pilgrimage as responses to plague. Instead, prayer, fasting and good behaviour were the ways religious people responded to plague in Protestant England.

Running away

Fear was a natural reaction to a plague epidemic. No-one understood how plague was spread, but everyone knew it was infectious and that it could kill you. It is not surprising, therefore, that many people tried to leave an infected town. Most aldermen and church ministers stayed out of a sense of duty, but running away from plague was an accepted response to the disease. In most cases, this was only an option for the wealthy who might have a house or friends in the country. The 'middling sort' and the labouring poor remained because they had nowhere else to go.

Reflect

What changes and continuities from the Middle Ages have you found so far?

▼ A seventeenth-century print showing people running away from the plague

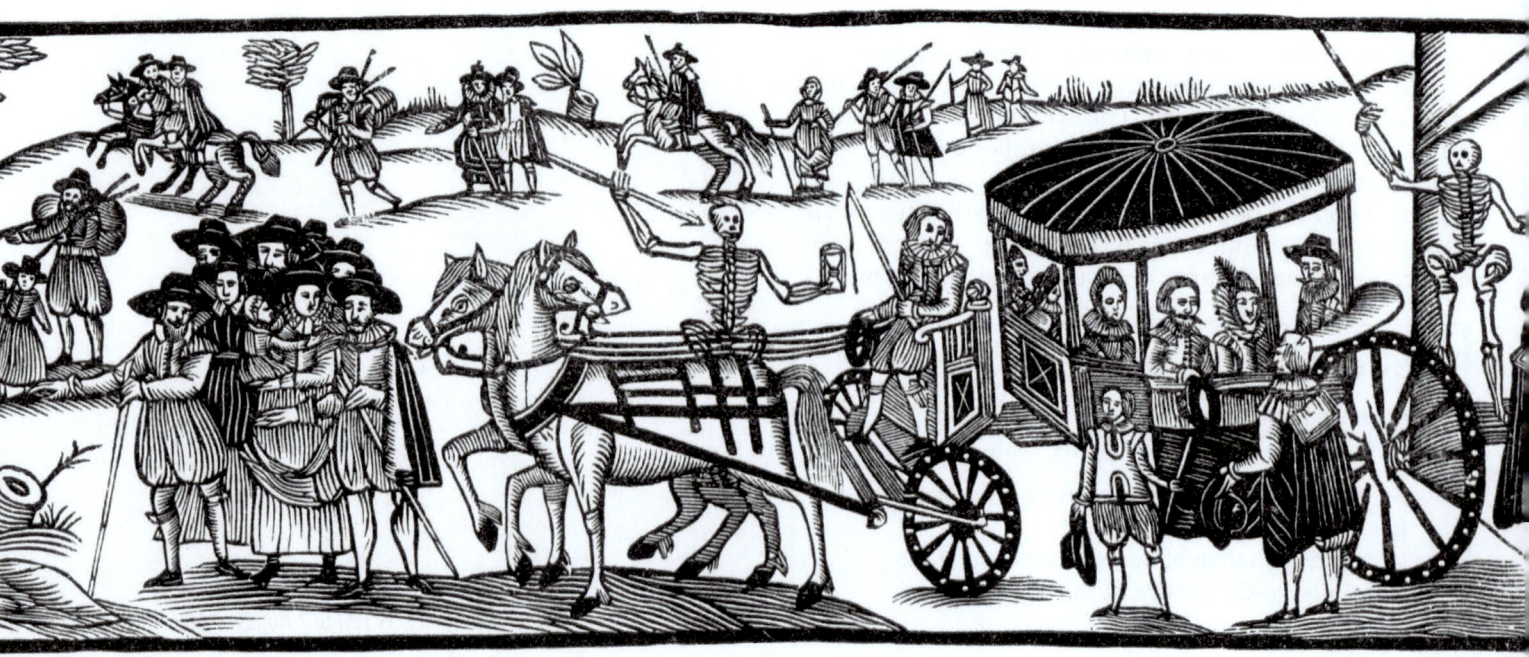

Seeking a cure

For those who remained in an infected town, the fear they must have faced is hard for us to imagine. People who caught the disease had little hope of receiving any medical treatment. From the later sixteenth century, physicians and apothecaries were becoming more common in English towns. Some physicians would treat those who could afford to pay, but many physicians fled. Those who stayed took the precaution of wearing heavy cloaks, hoods and leather beaks stuffed with sweet-smelling herbs. Apothecaries were often praised for staying rather than fleeing. People might buy tobacco as protection from miasma, or herbal remedies to ease their pain, but the shelves in the apothecary's shop contained nothing which could cure the plague.

Avoiding the sick

The threat of catching the disease placed people's relationships with neighbours, friends and family under huge strain. It is not surprising that people avoided the sick. People were understandably reluctant to take food to plague victims, to enter a house in order to write the will of a dying person, or to attend the funeral of a neighbour. The plague could have a negative impact of the relationship between masters and servants. Maids and apprentices were occasionally thrown out of their masters' houses and died on the streets. Some people looked for scapegoats whom they could blame for spreading the disease. Occasionally, there were violent attacks on individual foreigners and beggars.

Sticking together

Plague in early modern England certainly divided communities and sometimes led to bad behaviour. In general, however, communities did not collapse into panic and disorder. Violence directed at outsiders was rare. Few people abandoned members of their immediate family. Parents looked after their children. Husband and wives stayed together. The elderly took in orphaned children. Some people carried food and ale to their sick friends and neighbours. Many of the people who died had a dignified funeral attended by their friends and family.

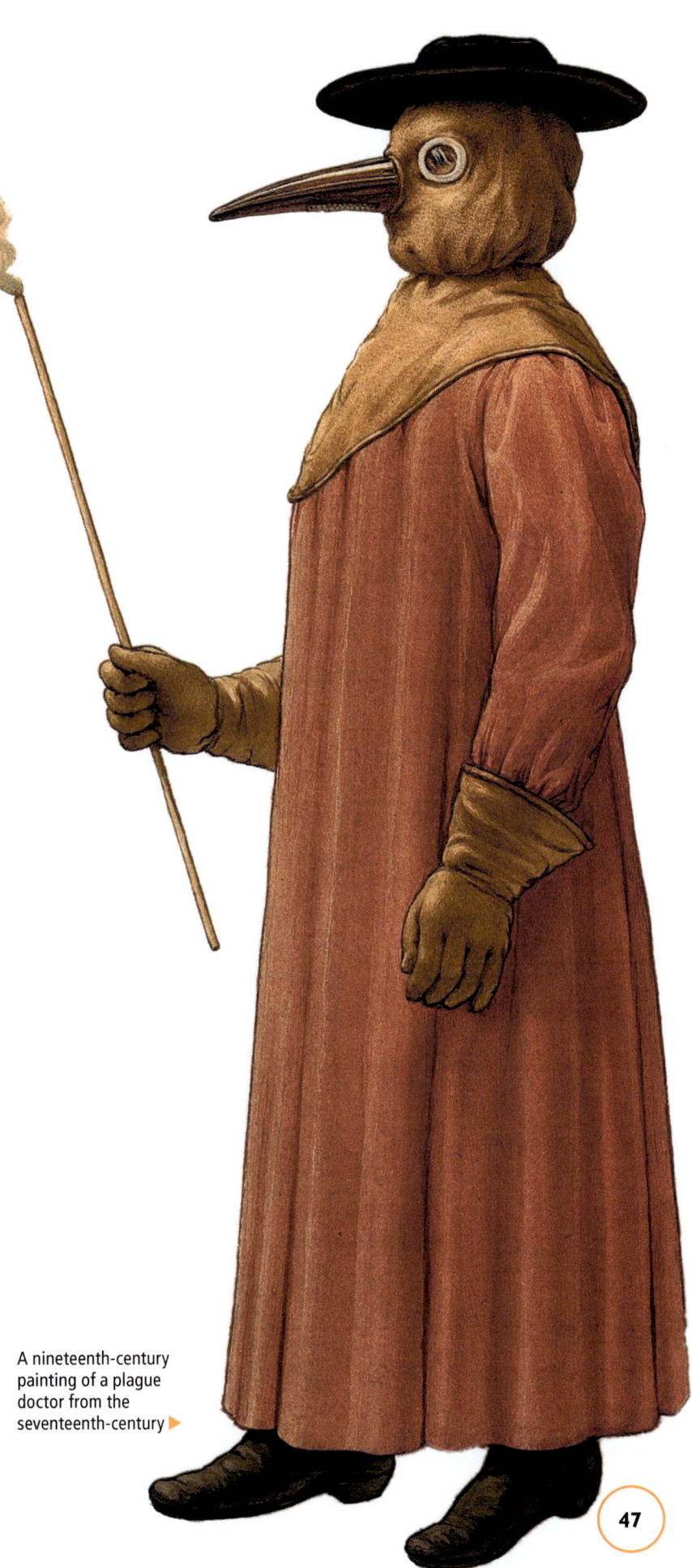

A nineteenth-century painting of a plague doctor from the seventeenth-century ▶

The impact of national and local government on public health

Record

This final section will help you to make up your mind about how far the authorities in early modern England improved public health. You will find out:

1. How councils tried to keep their towns clean in the period 1500–1670.
2. How much town life improved after plague disappeared, 1670–1750.
3. How the national government responded to a new threat to the people's health after 1660 – gin.

Summarise each section by writing five tweets. Make your first tweet a big idea or 'main point' and your next four tweets examples or 'supporting points'. Remember, each tweet can have no more than 140 characters, including spaces.

Filth and fines: the impact of local government on public health, 1500–1670

In the previous section (page 44) you found out how the national government began to issue plague orders to protect people's health. The plague orders of 1518, 1578 and 1604 were the first examples of a national policy on public health. You have seen how the government relied on local officials, particularly in the towns, to implement the measures at times of plague. Generally, mayors and aldermen did their best to isolate plague victims, to collect money for families who were shut up and to appoint watchmen and searchers. However, it was not only at times of plague that town corporations made efforts to keep their towns clean.

One historian who studied sixteenth-century records in York's archives made some interesting findings about public health in the city. York was the third largest and wealthiest city in England, after Norwich and London. The photograph below from around 1900 shows the Shambles, a street in the centre of York that had changed very little since the sixteenth century. It was where butchers sold meat from their open-fronted shops in the sixteenth century. The buildings and the line of the street had changed very little since the sixteenth century. Around the photograph are some of the rules which York's aldermen enforced in the 1500s.

Pigs had to be kept in a sty and were not allowed to wander around the streets.

Household waste could not be put out for the scavengers until 7pm.

If your cesspit was overflowing you could pay for the scavengers who would clean it out for you.

Anyone who made a dunghill in their yard had to pay a fine.

People were fined for throwing urine and excrement into the street at night.

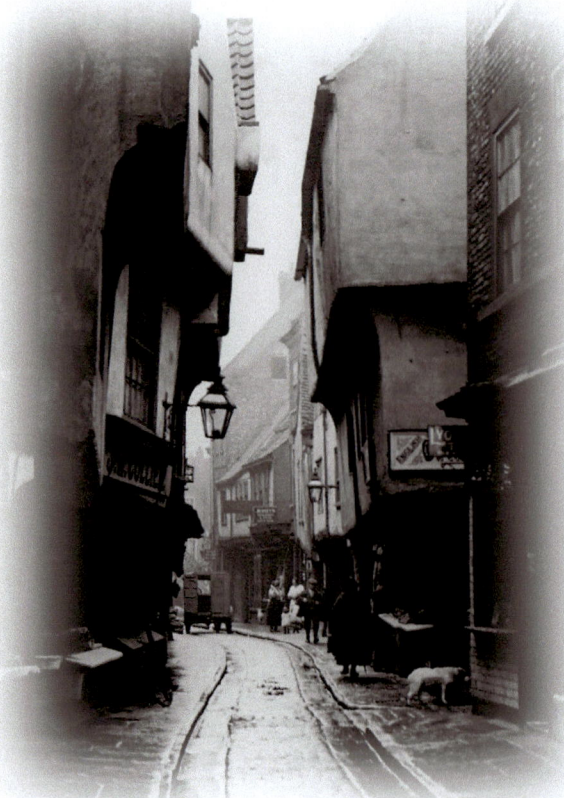

People were not allowed to build their privies over the Queen's Dike, a stream which ran through the city.

All householders had to clean the street outside their property twice a week.

Nobody could block the gutters which ran down both sides of York's main streets.

Record

Write your five tweets about how the aldermen of York tried to keep their town clean. Remember to make your first tweet a big idea about public health in sixteenth-century York. How does this compare with what you know about public health in medieval towns?

◀ The Shambles, York, c.1900

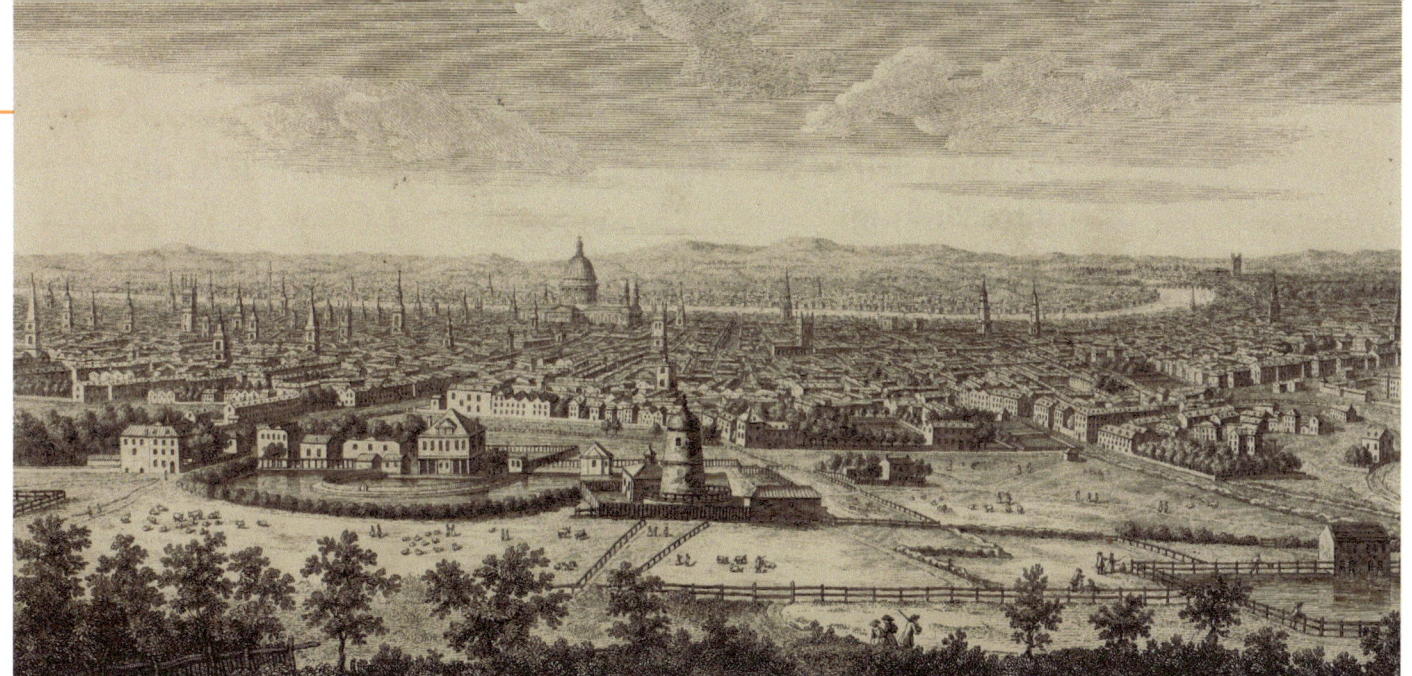

▲ Panorama of London from the north, 1752

Room for improvement: the impact of local government on public health, 1670–1750

After 1670, town corporations no longer had to worry about dealing with outbreaks of plague. Instead they could concentrate on improving the urban environment in order to make towns more pleasant places in which to live. This print of London was made in 1752. It gives us a view of the city from the north, nearly 150 years after the panorama that we began with on pages 30–31. You can see the dome of St Paul's cathedral, built by Christopher Wren after the Great Fire of London in 1666. The spires of some of Wren's other churches are dotted around the city. In the middle of the picture is the reservoir that Hugh Middleton had built in 1609 to bring water into London. Nearby was a yard where tree trunks of elm trees were bored to make water pipes. By 1750, several water companies in London and in other towns piped water into the homes of those who could afford an annual subscription.

In the period 1670–1750, local authorities made big improvements to the centres of their towns in order to cope with the growing number of people, carriages and carts. Many councils encouraged builders to construct streets and squares of large terraced houses where wealthy people could live. This 1750 print of Fenchurch Street in the centre of London gives you an idea of the kinds of improvements which were made. Many more streets were now paved with stone, and lines of posts marked off footways for pedestrians. Oil-burning street lamps first appeared in London in the 1680s and by 1750 most towns had lighting in their main streets.

Town councils made these improvements because they wanted to make town life more pleasant. The people's health was certainly not their main concern. In the period before 1750, the connection between dirt and disease had not yet been made. There was a big contrast between the improved areas and the poorer neighbourhoods where streets were unpaved and unlit, and where people still had to fetch water from a public conduit or buy it from a water cart. For everyone, sewage disposal had hardly improved since the 1660s when Samuel Pepys had stepped in his neighbour's turds. It would be another hundred years before sewers removed the problem of stinking, overflowing cesspits.

Record

Write your five tweets about the impact of local government on public health 1670–1750. Make your first tweet a 'main point' about how much town life improved.

▼ An engraving of Fenchurch Street, c.1750

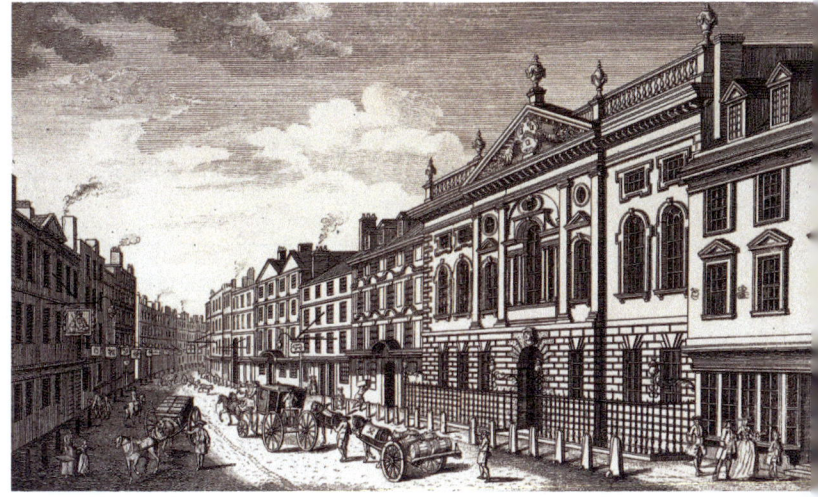

Demon drink: the impact of national government on gin drinking

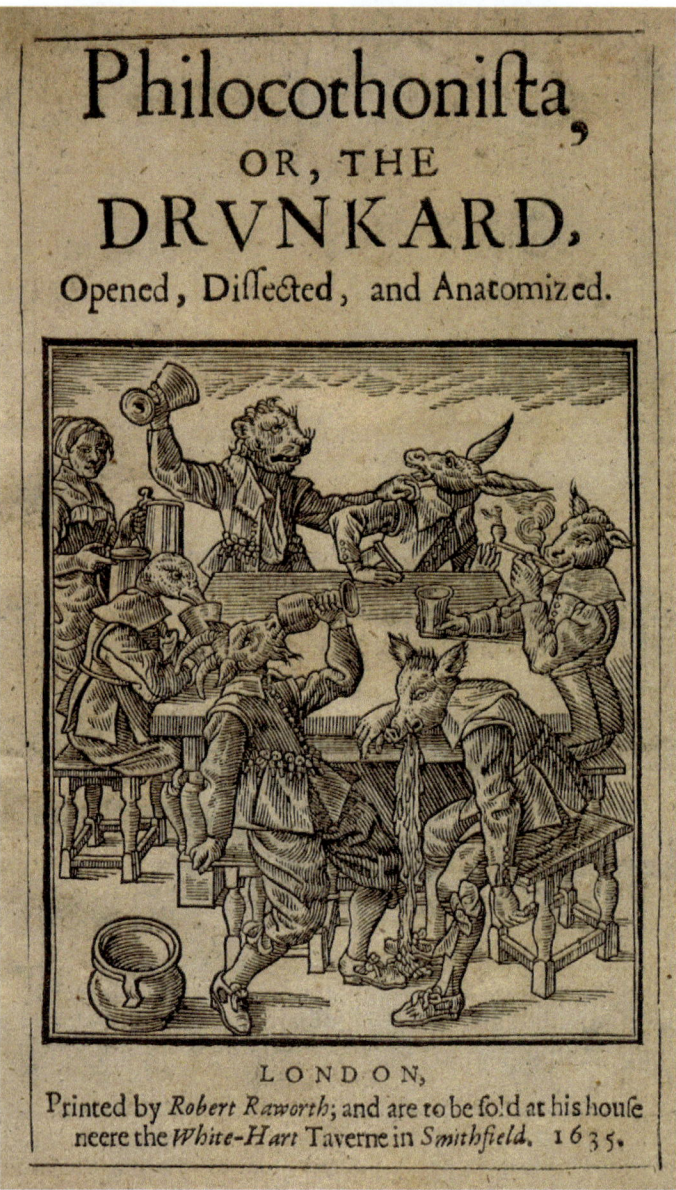

Ale and beer drinking had been widespread in England since the Middle Ages. In the early modern period, there was a huge growth in the number of alehouses and drunkenness became a real problem. Puritans, in particular, were concerned about drunkenness and wrote pamphlets attacking the demon drink. From around 1550, town councils and county justices tried to control alehouses by making it illegal to sell alcohol without a licence. By the 1630s, measures to control alehouses and drunkenness had begun to have a real impact in many towns and villages. It did not last.

After 1660, alcohol became a big problem for people's health because many poor people started drinking spirits rather than ale or beer. This was a particular issue in London where many 'dram shops' opened, selling cheap spirits such as brandy and gin. At first gin was imported from Holland where it was first produced in the 1650s. In 1689, parliament banned imports of gin in order to encourage distillers in England. Gin became incredibly cheap and there was a huge increase in gin drinking by London's poor. Thousands of small 'gin shops' opened in cellars, back rooms, attics and sheds. Some people even sold it from barrows in the streets.

By the 1720s, gin had become a big social and health problem in London. Hundreds of thousands of poor men and women turned to gin as an escape from the misery of lack of work and poor living conditions. Gin shops advertised 'drunk for a penny, dead drunk for two pence'. Crime went up, families were ruined and there was a huge increase in the death rate. In 1729, parliament finally made a law to control gin drinking. Gin distillers had to pay a tax of five shillings on each gallon of gin they produced and gin sellers had to buy an annual licence costing £20. The new law had little effect – it was impossible to enforce the 1729 Gin Act because there were so many small gin shops.

In 1736, the government passed a harsher Gin Act. Licences went up to £50 and the tax was increased to twenty shillings. Again, the act could not be enforced. It was too easy for the gin shops to hide what they were doing from the authorities. In 1743, parliament tried something else. The 1743 Gin Act restricted the sale of gin to alehouses which already sold ale, beer and wine. Gin consumption still continued to increase. By 1750, Londoners were consuming over 11 million gallons of gin a year.

> ### Reflect
> This picture from a pamphlet attacking drunkards was printed in 1635. How does the picture portray the effects of alcohol? Can you spot a connection with the picture of drunkards on page 13?

In 1751, the government finally introduced a law which had an effect on gin drinking. The Gin Act of 1751 was much tougher than any of the previous acts in 1729, 1736 and 1743. Anyone caught selling gin illegally was imprisoned and whipped for a second offence. A third offence could result in transportation. Gin drinking was hugely reduced. At last, the national government had got to grips with this major problem affecting the people's health.

More of the same?

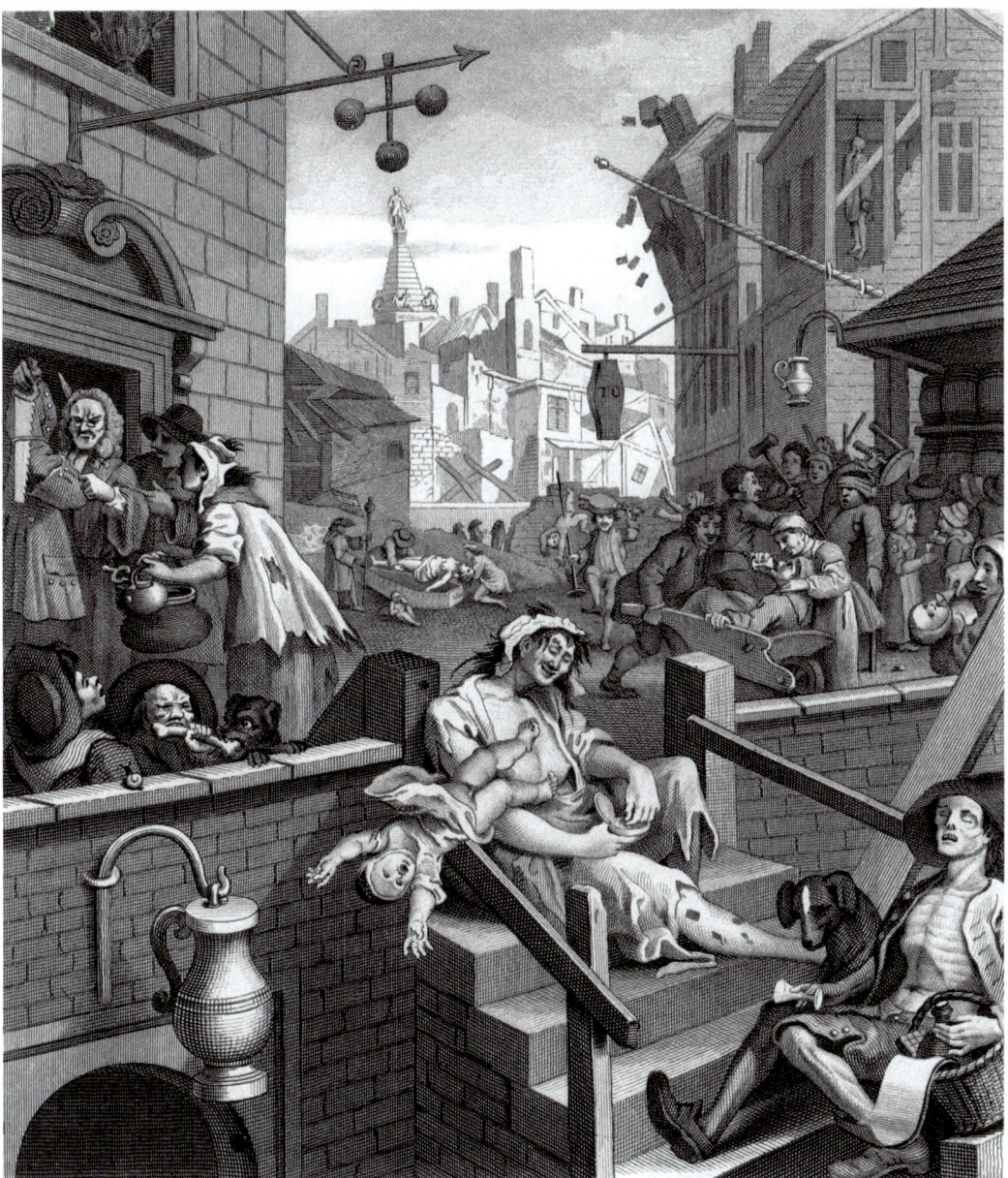

◀ The artist William Hogarth was a strong critic of the gin trade. In 1751, he produced his engraving 'Gin Lane' which gave a realistic and horrifying picture of the evils of gin

Reflect
What details did Hogarth include in his engraving to show the horrors of the gin trade?

Record
Write your five tweets about how the national government introduced measures to control gin drinking.

Review
In this enquiry you have produced clear and detailed notes on three issues relating the people's health in the period 1500–1750: living conditions, plague and the impact of local and national government on public health.

Use your notes to make up your mind about how much people's health changed in the period 1500–1750. For each of the three issues you have studied, place an 'X' somewhere on a continuum like the one below to show how much change you think there had been. Underneath the continuum, write a clear, organised and detailed explanation to support your judgement.

A lot of change ——————————————————— Very little change

CLOSER LOOK 2

The 1636 plague in Newcastle

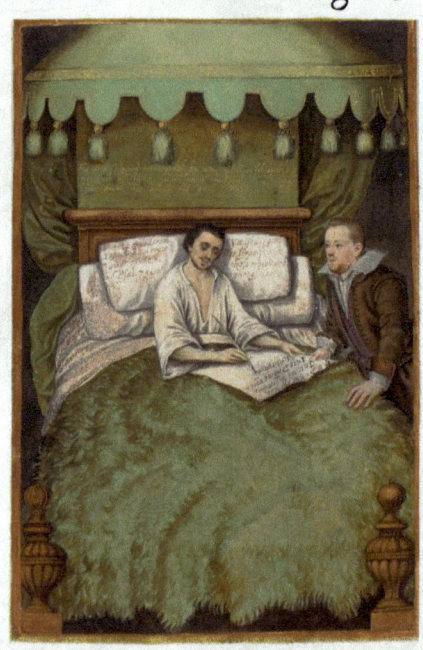

▲ The cover of Keith Wrightson's book, *Ralph Tailor's Summer, A Scrivener, his City and the Plague*

▼ A map of Newcastle in 1636

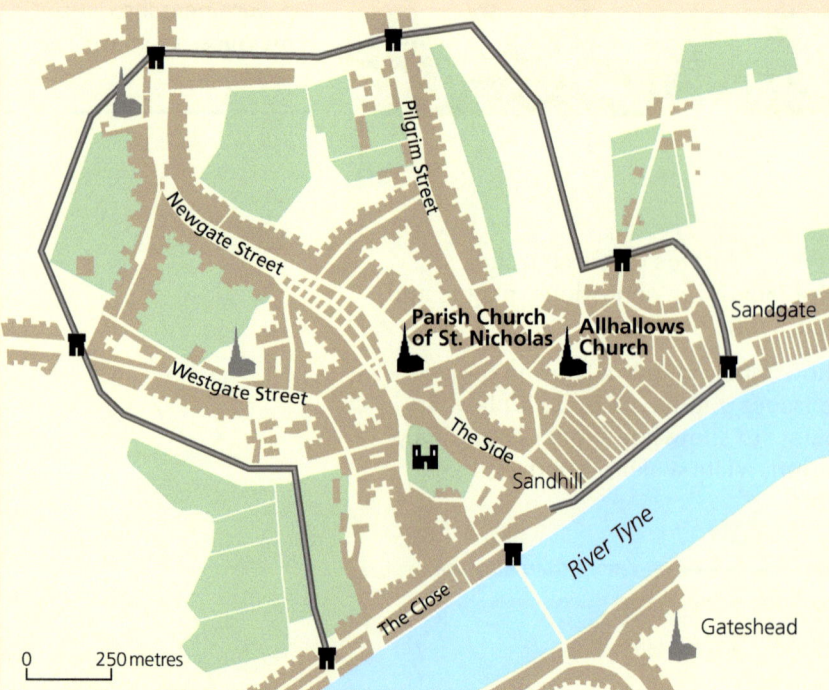

Sometimes in history it helps to zoom in *really* close. One day, when working on some dusty documents from seventeenth-century Newcastle, the historian Keith Wrightson came across several wills written by the same man – Ralph Tailor. Ralph was a twenty-five-year-old scrivener. He made his living by writing documents for people in Newcastle. In the summer of 1636, many people in the city needed Ralph Tailor to write their wills because Newcastle was in the grip of a plague epidemic. Keith Wrightson became fascinated by the 1636 plague in Newcastle. He made a careful study of all the documents written by Ralph Tailor and extended his research to other sources. Professor Wrightson hoped that by making a detailed study of Newcastle in 1636 he could gain a deeper understanding of the impact of plague in early modern England, and of how people responded to this devastating threat to their families and community.

With a population of 12,000, Newcastle was the fifth largest city in England in the 1630s. Situated on the side of a steep hill on the north side of the River Tyne, Newcastle was a rich and beautiful city. Its wealth came from trade with Europe and from shipping coal down the English coast to London. In the seventeenth century, Newcastle's wealthiest inhabitants lived in the central part of the city along the wide streets leading to the parish church of St Nicholas. The poorer people crowded into the narrow lanes which ran from Allhallows Church down to the river. Just outside the city walls there was a particularly poor area called Sandgate where Newcastle's public dunghill was located. Here, a large number of people lived by the quayside in cramped houses infested with rats.

At the beginning of May 1636, people in Sandgate began to die of plague. During the summer, as the disease spread across Newcastle, the number of deaths rose every week. By August, over 300 people a week were buried in the city's churchyards. In October, the plague began to retreat, but in five months it had killed at least 5,600 people, 47 per cent of Newcastle's population. Such a high mortality was catastrophic for the city as a whole, but in the poorer districts, where the death rate was even higher, the disease must have been devastating.

The 1636 plague in Newcastle

Professor Wrightson found that few records had survived which could reveal exactly how Newcastle's corporation responded to the 1636 plague, but he was able to piece together the basic story. Newcastle's mayor and aldermen paid careful attention to the national plague orders. They appointed 'searchers' to report plague deaths, organised the burials of the dead, ensured that tar barrels were burned in the streets and provided food for people living in poverty who could no longer work. The corporation also enforced a strict quarantine, shutting up plague victims in their houses and isolating some of the sick in 'lodges' on the town moor to the north of the city. Overall, Keith Wrightson felt that Newcastle's leaders rose to the challenge of responding to the plague.

▼ A will written by Ralph Tailor

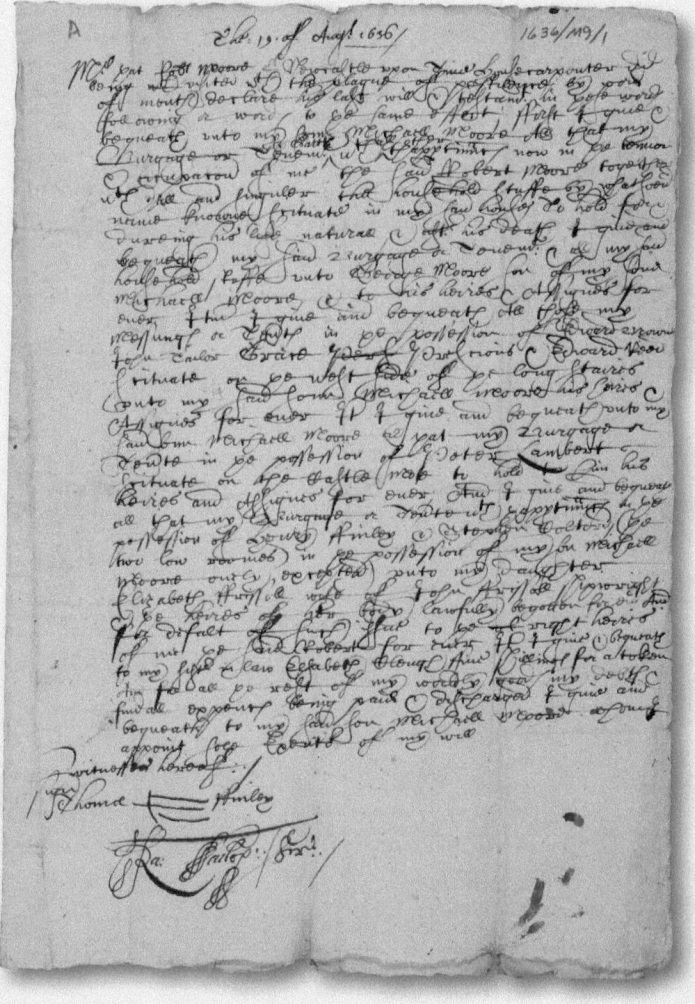

▼ Sellar's Entry in Sandgate, c.1895

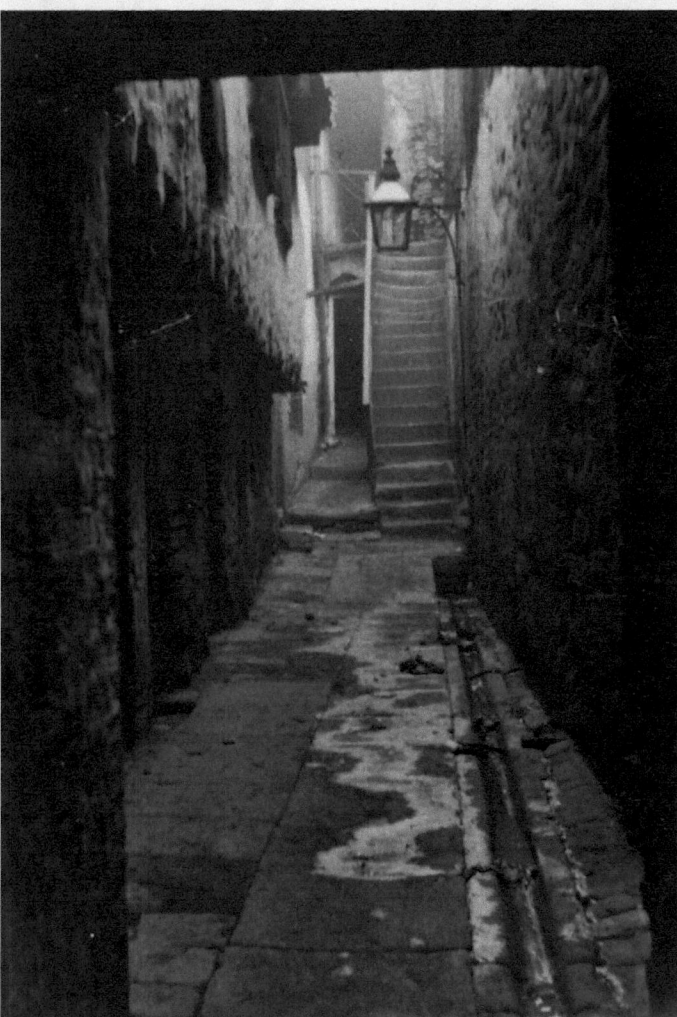

As the plague raged in Newcastle through the summer of 1636, Ralph Tailor was kept very busy writing wills for the dying. Many of these were in the parish of Allhallows where Ralph bravely visited people in their shut up houses. Newcastle's wealthier inhabitants left the city if they could and went to live in the country, but most people could not flee as they had nowhere to go. Professor Wrightson discovered that the ordinary people left in the city often tried their best to help the sick and dying. He found very few references to doctors visiting the sick, but discovered that many poor women were hired as 'keepers' to look after families shut up in their houses. Many people risked their own lives to act as witnesses to wills, to take food and drink to the sick, to attend funerals and to take in plague victims who had no one to care for them. During the plague of 1636, the people of Newcastle controlled their fear and did not give up on each other.

3 Revolution!

Why were there such huge changes in the people's health, 1750–1900?

The engraving below shows Manchester's River Irwell in the middle of the nineteenth century. In 1750, Manchester was a small town with a population of 17,000. By 1850, it was a gigantic industrial city containing a third of a million people. Life in early nineteenth-century Manchester was grim. The factory chimneys poured out thick smoke which hung heavily over the city. An absence of sunlight led to vitamin deficiencies which caused many people to suffer from rickets. In the factories, the air pollution and frequent accidents shortened people's lives. Manchester's mill workers lived in damp, dirty and overcrowded houses where diseases such as tuberculosis and typhus flourished. As more and more people moved into Manchester, the existing water supplies and sewers could not cope with demand. Families struggled to obtain clean water. Sewage festered in cesspools, stood in dunghills or found its way into the River Irwell. Huge numbers of people died of water-borne diseases. In 1841, average life expectancy in Manchester was just 26.6 years.

Cholera

James Palfreyman was a healthy 29-year-old man who worked as a coach painter in Manchester in 1832. His wages were slightly higher than those of the mill workers and he could afford to live in one of the better streets in the city. On the evening of

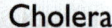
An engraving of the River Irwell in Manchester, 1867

Why were there such huge changes in the people's health, 1750–1900?

Tuesday 15 May, James drank too much beer in his local pub. The next day he went to work. For his main meal of the day he ate a plateful of lamb's head, liver, lungs and heart. This would be James' last meal. On the Thursday, he was too unwell to go to work. He started to vomit and had terrible stomach cramps. James suffered vomiting and diarrhoea for two days. On Saturday 19 May 1832, at 2.30 p.m., he died. James Palfreyman was the first person to die of cholera in Manchester. This dreadful disease had first appeared in Britain in October 1831. It spread quickly, killing 31,000 people in England and Scotland by the autumn of 1832. A second outbreak in 1848 was even worse – this time, 65,000 people died.

Improvements

Cholera returned to Britain again in 1853 and 1866, but killed fewer people. The first cholera outbreaks of 1831 and 1848 had shocked national and local government into action. At first, no one knew that cholera was spread by germs in people's drinking water, but many people were convinced that the disease flourished in dirty living conditions. They argued that a big clean-up was needed and began to campaign for improvements to public health. During the second half of the nineteenth century, the authorities made efforts to provide people with clean water and proper sewerage.

By 1900, the public health crisis which Britain had experienced in the first part of the nineteenth century was a distant memory. The work of some remarkable individuals, combined with a range of other factors, meant that the people's health had finally begun to improve.

The Enquiry

As you have just discovered, there were huge changes in the people's health in the period 1750–1900:

- In the first part of the nineteenth century, industrialisation and urbanisation created a public health crisis in Britain.
- An outbreak of cholera in 1831–32 killed thousands of people, created fear and shocked the authorities into action.
- From the 1830s, public health campaigns led to some big improvements in the people's health.

In this enquiry your challenge is to analyse these three changes, and to explain why each occurred.

As in the previous two enquiries, it will be useful to begin with an overview of some of the big changes in Britain during this period …

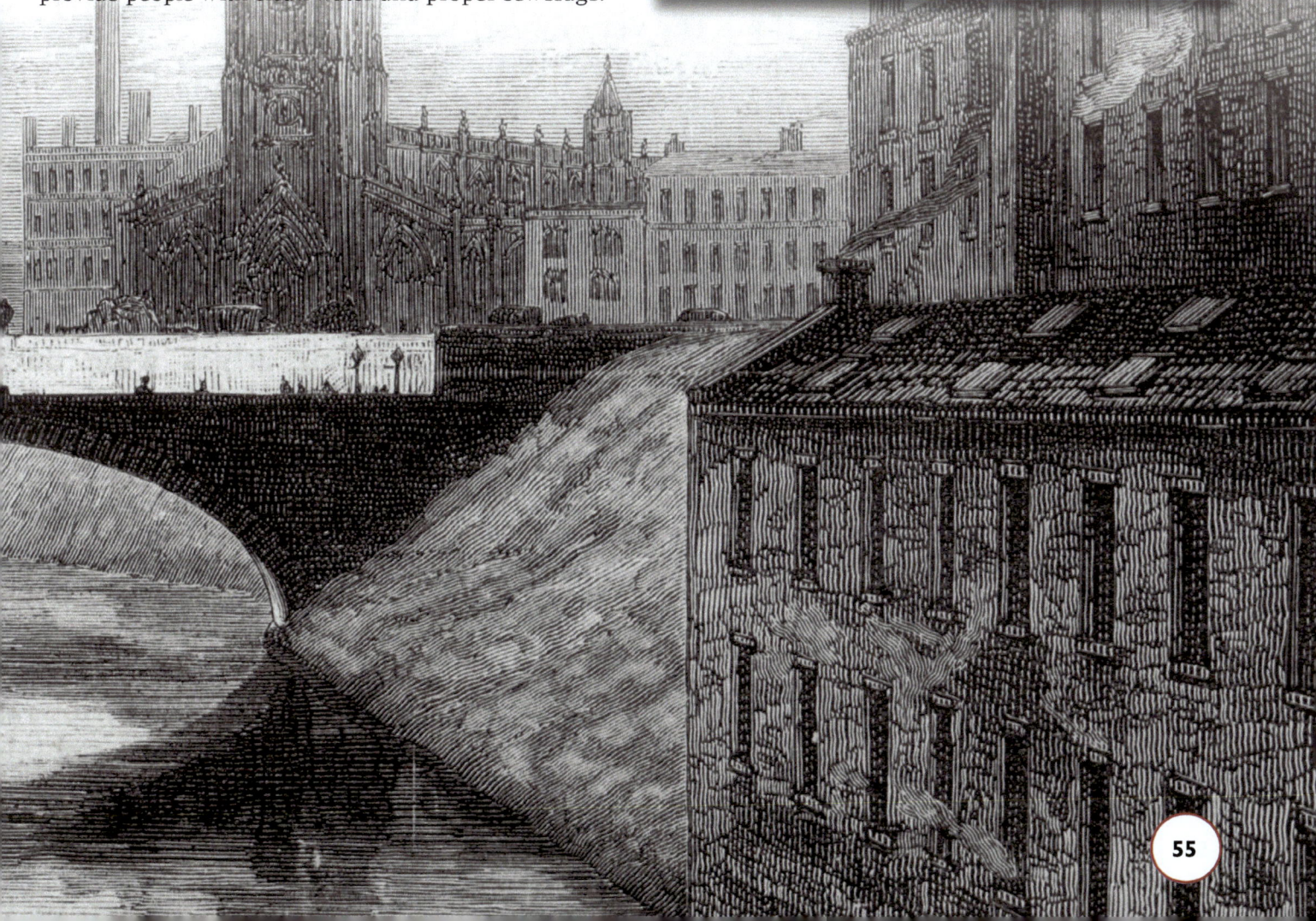

Britain 1750–1900: an overview

> **Record**
>
> The next four pages summarise different aspects of life in Britain, 1750–1900. Read through them quickly and make a list of at least six specific features that you think may have affected people's health at that time. Collect and explain your ideas in a table like this one:
>
> | Specific feature of life at this time | How I think this may have affected the people's health |
> |---|---|
> | | |

1. Food supply

After 1750, Britain's population rocketed – from around 6 million in 1750, it grew to 21 million in 1850, and to 37 million by 1900. Improvements in agriculture, like the introduction of new machinery, meant that Britain's growing population did not starve. However, the wages of labouring families were too low to provide an adequate diet. George Mitchell, who was brought up in a labouring family in Somerset during the 1830s, was sometimes so hungry that he ate turnips from the fields and collected snails to roast for his tea. In the cities, poorer people found it difficult to obtain fresh and safe food. Sometimes, all they could afford to buy from the butcher were cheap cuts of meat from diseased animals.

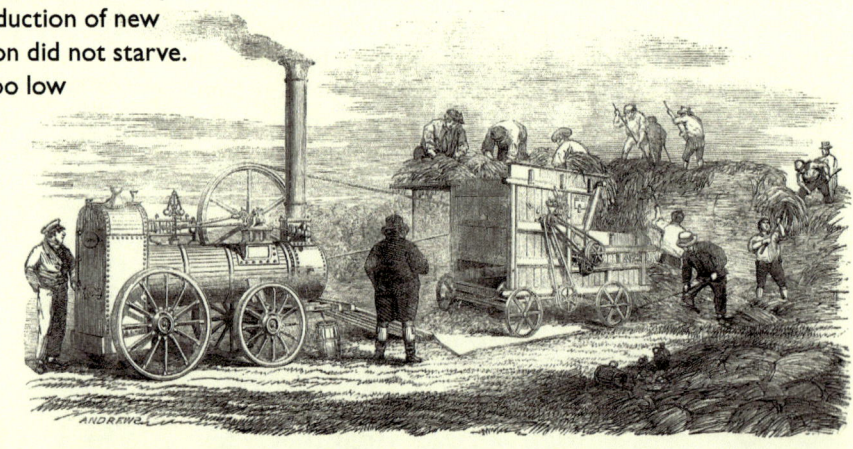

▼ Threshing by steam. An engraving from the late nineteenth century

2. Industrialisation

In the period 1750–1850, industrialisation transformed Britain. The first textile mills were powered by water, but by the early nineteenth century steam engines had improved to the point where they could be used to power machinery. The demand for coal increased, new mines opened and canals were built to transport the coal to the factories. In Manchester, and in other industrial cities, hundreds of factory chimneys belched out smoke, creating a thick smog over the streets. As Britain's towns and cities expanded, more and more people also used cheap coal in their houses. The smoke from their chimney pots added to the air pollution from the factories. In London, the fumes from hundreds of breweries, potteries, glass-makers and other manufacturers combined with the smoke from houses to create thick 'pea-souper' fogs.

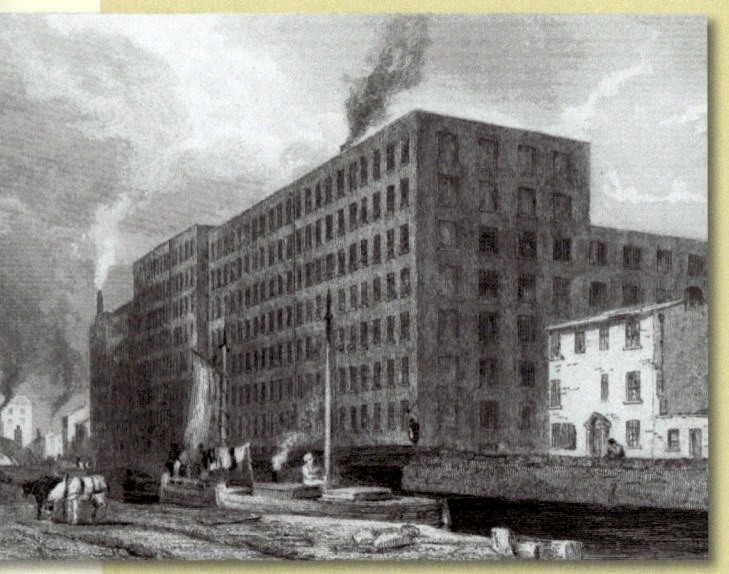

◀ A steam-powered cotton mill in Manchester in 1835

Why were there such huge changes in the people's health, 1750–1900?

3. Working conditions

This picture, from 1835, shows the interior of a textile mill in the north of England. The picture portrays a textile factory in a very positive light. The sun shines through the windows. The female workers look well-dressed, clean and healthy. But the reality of factory work was quite different. In the early nineteenth century, children working in Manchester's factories started at 5 a.m., had half an hour for breakfast, half an hour for lunch and finished work at 6 p.m. Hour after hour, they breathed in the dusty air of the factory. The noise from the machinery was deafening and accidents were common.

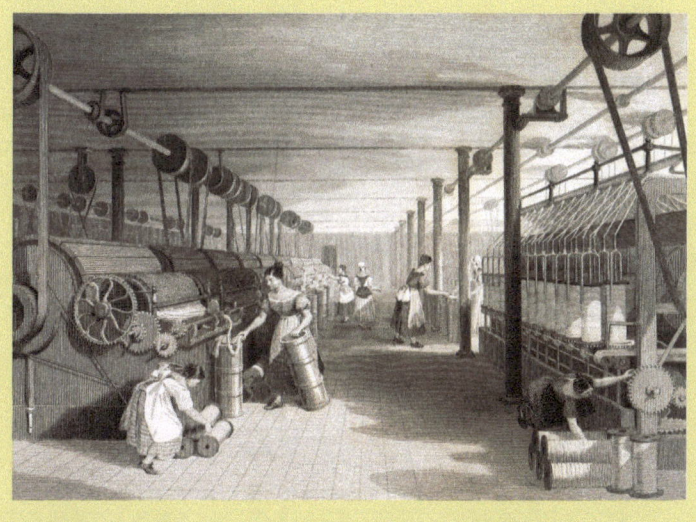

▶ Workers in a textile factory in 1835

4. The British Empire

In 1750, Britain was already an important trading nation with colonies in America and the Caribbean. The American colonies became independent in 1783, but Britain expanded its empire in other parts of the world, particularly in India. This map shows the extent of the British Empire in 1886 (Britain's territories are coloured pink). By the end of the nineteenth century, much of Africa was also under British control. In 1900, Britain ruled one-fifth of the world's land and a quarter of the world's population. Over the period 1750 to 1900, the huge growth in trade across the British Empire brought new plants, animals, foods, ideas and diseases to Britain, though this was often at great cost to the parts of the world that the British colonised.

◀ A map of the British Empire, 1886

5. Urbanisation and the railways

In this engraving, the French artist Gustave Doré gives us a glimpse of London in 1870. In the period 1750–1900, it was not just the new industrial towns and cities which experienced rapid growth. London, and other older urban centres, also expanded. Living conditions varied between towns, but everywhere such rapid growth placed huge pressures on the urban environment. Doré illustrates the overcrowding and the difficulties of water supply in this part of London. His engraving also includes a new development in nineteenth-century Britain – railways. The first inter-city railway in the world opened between Liverpool and Manchester in 1830. By 1850, a network of railways covered many parts of Britain. Railways brought fresh food to the towns and allowed people to escape to the countryside and coast. But they also added to the pollution of the urban environment.

▼ 'London back yards from a train', Gustave Doré, 1870

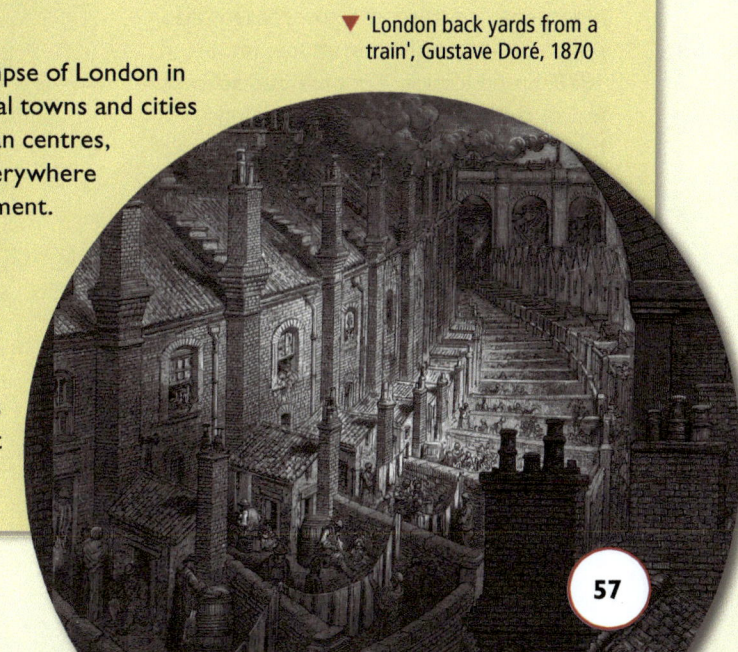

6. Changing beliefs

In the period 1750–1900, many people were influenced by new scientific thinking which challenged religious views. In 1859, the man in this photograph, Charles Darwin, published his book on evolution, *The Origin of the Species*. Darwin's theory of evolution challenged the story of creation found in the Bible. It led to a huge shift in the way people understood the world. By the end of the nineteenth century, many people in Britain believed that science had disproved Christianity. For centuries religion had governed people's view of the world, but by 1900 Britain was becoming a secular society.

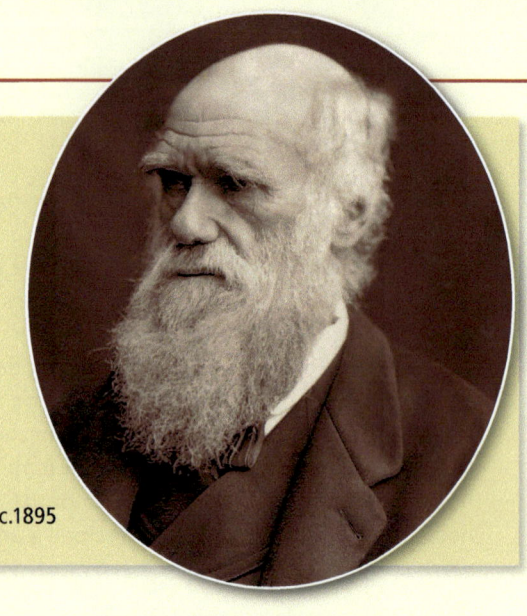

▶ Charles Darwin, c.1895

7. New discoveries

The man looking through his microscope in this painting is the French scientist Louis Pasteur. In 1861, Pasteur made one of the most important discoveries in human history – that harmful germs could enter the human body, grow fast and cause disease. In the late nineteenth century, other scientists built on Pasteur's work by identifying the individual germs which caused specific diseases. At last, in 1861, the true cause of human disease had been discovered!

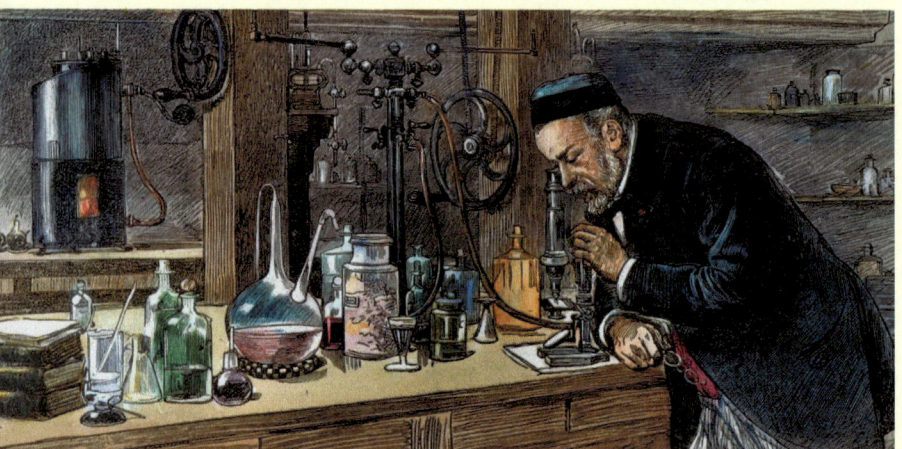

◀ Louis Pasteur in his laboratory

8. Growing literacy

In 1750, few children in Britain went to school but, in the late eighteenth century, charities and churches began to provide schools for poorer children. During the nineteenth century, the government also began to get involved in education. In 1870, an Education Act provided schools for all children under the age of ten. Improvements in education meant that more people could read and this fuelled a growth in demand for newspapers. Daily and weekly newspapers began to play an important part in people's lives as more and more people enjoyed reading about sporting events, crimes, politics and other matters. By the end of the century, many newspapers were illustrated and contained advertisements like the ones shown here.

▼ Illustrated advertisements from a late-nineteenth-century newspaper

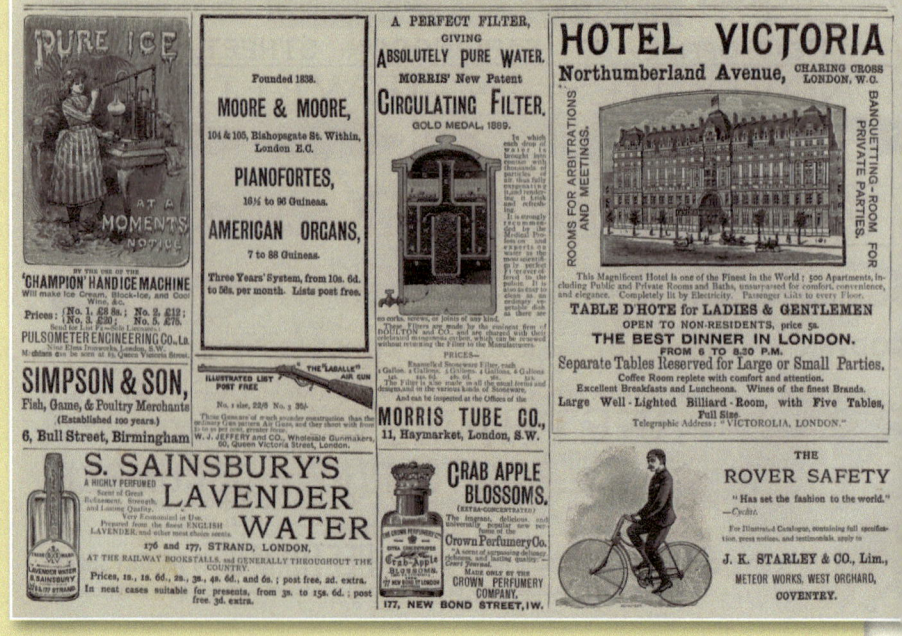

9. The growth of democracy

Until 1832, only 5 per cent of the population could vote in elections for the House of Commons and no women were allowed to vote. Few of Britain's new industrial cities were represented by their own members of parliament. Change came with the 1832 Reform Act which gave the vote to men who owned property and allowed the larger towns to have two MPs each. In 1867 and 1884, the vote was extended to working-class men. During the nineteenth century, national and local government began to play a bigger part in people's lives. By the end of the century it had become quite normal for the government to pass laws which tried to improve the lives of poorer people.

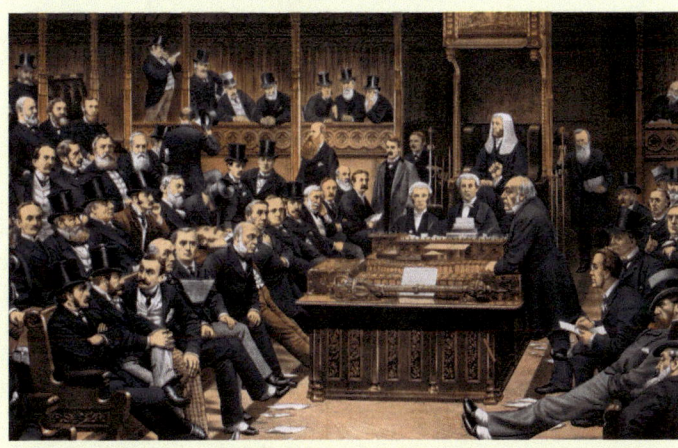

A debate in the House of Commons, 1887

10. Class divisions

In his 1888 painting *Poverty and Wealth,* the artist William Powell Frith depicted the inequality in Victorian Britain. On the left, a wealthy family sit in their carriage in a London street. They are watched by a group of poor people on the right of the picture. In the nineteenth century, factory-owners and professional people moved out of the centres of industrial towns and cities. They built spacious villas in the clean air and pleasant surroundings of the suburbs and countryside. In contrast, working-class people crowded into the slums of the city centres to be close to the factories where they worked. Few middle-class people ever ventured into poor, working-class districts. Most of them remained ignorant about the living conditions and daily struggles of people living in poverty.

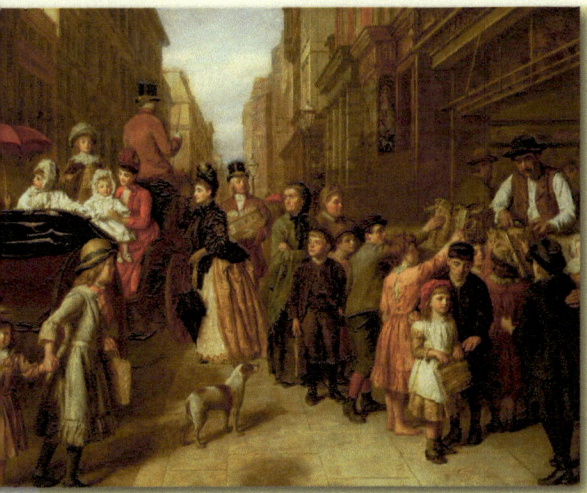

◀ 'Poverty and Wealth' by William Powell Frith, 1888

11. Alcohol

People in industrial Britain drank too much. The middle classes enjoyed a bottle of wine with their dinner, and many wealthier men drank large quantities of brandy and port. Working-class people also consumed too much alcohol, but they drank in the pub rather than in the home. The pub provided a warm, well-lit and pleasant escape from the slums. Some poorer people became addicted to alcohol and drank huge quantities of beer and whisky. Gin, too, remained a problem, even after the end of the 'gin craze' in 1751. Drunkenness became such an issue in the nineteenth century that a 'Temperance Movement' was formed which tried to persuade people to stop drinking alcohol. It had limited success.

▼ A crowded pub in the East End of London, 1871

Dirty towns: the public health crisis in early industrial Britain

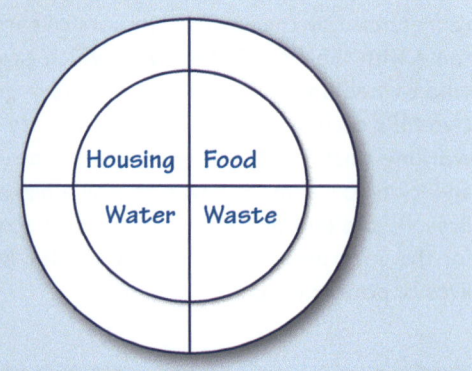

Record

As you find out about the public health crisis in the first part of the nineteenth century, use a big version of the diagram opposite to collect your ideas. In the centre circle, summarise the unhealthy conditions under the headings: housing, food, water and waste. In the outer circle, explain the reasons for the public health crisis.

The early industrial towns of the North and Midlands were grim places. One visitor to Leeds in 1848 described the city as 'a perfect wilderness of foulness'. Industrial workers often lived in cramped, squalid houses close to the factories where they worked. Few had running water and hardly any were connected to sewers. Often, several families shared a single privy. Human waste collected in cesspools and overflowed into the yards and streets. Killer diseases such as tuberculosis, typhoid and diphtheria were common. In 1842, 57 per cent of children born in the working-class districts of Manchester died before the age of five. There were five main reasons for these terrible living conditions in the first half of the nineteenth century:

1. **Towns and cities grew incredibly quickly**

   From the end of the eighteenth century when the Industrial Revolution took off, people poured into the urban areas. The existing infrastructure of the towns just could not cope with the increase in numbers.

2. **The supply of houses could not keep up with demand**

   Landlords could make big profits from renting homes to industrial workers. They built houses quickly and cheaply. Many property-owners and builders showed little concern for the quality of housing.

3. **Town government was weak**

   Many expanding towns did not have a corporation and were governed by several different authorities. Many of the property-owners who governed the towns did not want an increase in their rates (local taxes) in order to provide clean water and sewers for people living in poverty.

4. **There were no laws to ensure decent housing and to protect people's health**

   National and local government had a *laissez-faire* attitude, a belief that it was best not to not interfere in people's lives.

5. **People did not yet know that germs caused disease**

   It was not until after 1850 that people began to make a direct connection between dirty water and disease. Pasteur did not publish his germ theory until 1861 and it was not widely accepted until later in the nineteenth century.

Housing

All large towns in early industrial Britain had lodging houses where single people lived, and where newly-arrived families sometimes stayed while they looked for houses to rent. Lodging houses were often large, old houses divided up into smaller rooms. They varied a lot, but many were filthy and overcrowded. People were often packed into small rooms, sometimes sleeping on the floor or sharing a bed. In these conditions, disease spread quickly. Typhus (passed on by body lice) was common.

The best kind of dwelling a family could hope for was a through house, with its own back yard. Many people had to make do with a back-to-back house. Builders built these in order to pack as many houses as possible onto a small plot of land. Back-to-back terraces were built in double rows. Each house had its own front wall, but was joined to others at the back and sides.

Why were there such huge changes in the people's health, 1750–1900?

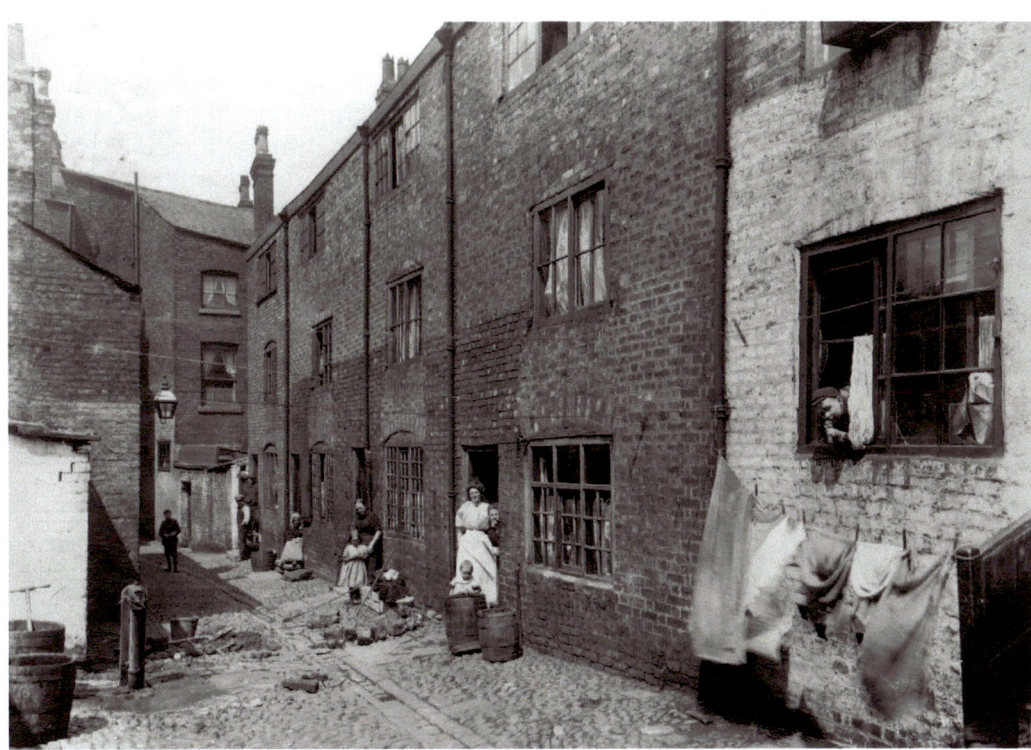

◀ A photograph of a Manchester yard, 1896

> **Reflect**
>
> Photography had only just been invented in the 1840s so there are hardly any photographs of the poor housing that existed at this time. This photograph of a Manchester yard was taken in 1896. What can it tell us about the living conditions of people living in poverty?

Some large families lived in back-to-back houses with just one room downstairs and another upstairs. It was particularly difficult to ventilate back-to-back houses and people who lived in them often suffered from chest infections and killer diseases like tuberculosis. Often, back-to-back houses were built around courts or yards, entered through a narrow alley from a main street.

Some of the very poorest people could not afford to rent even a back-to-back house in a street in a court. Instead, they crowded below ground in the cellars of other people's houses.

> **The Leeds surgeon, Robert Baker, described a cellar dwelling which he visited in 1842**
>
> I have been to one of these damp cellars, without the slightest drainage and every morsel of dirt and filth having to be carried up into the street; two corded frames for beds, overlaid with sacks for five persons; scarcely anything in the room to sit on, but a stool or a few bricks; the floor in many places absolutely wet; a pig in the corner also; and in a street where filth of all kinds has accumulated for years.

> **Reflect**
>
> What made cellar dwellings so unhealthy?

Food

People's poor diet played a major part in the public health crisis of the early nineteenth century. Industrial workers were cut off from the land and it was impossible to grow food in the slum districts of towns and cities. Working-class families were forced to buy their food from small shops and street-sellers. The incomes of many families were simply too low to buy sufficient food, particularly when there were several children to feed. Poor families lived mainly on bread, butter, potatoes and tea. Occasionally, cheap bacon, rabbit or offal provided a treat for better-off labouring families. As a result of their poor diet, many people in early industrial Britain were malnourished, making them prone to sickness and disease.

It was not only the *lack* of food which affected people's health in the early industrial towns – the *quality* of food was also an issue. Not until the 1860s was food preserved in cans. Refrigerators were not invented until the 1880s. In addition, the *laissez-faire* attitude meant that national and local government made little attempt to control the production and sale of food until the later nineteenth century. As a result, much of the food eaten by poor, urban workers was adulterated: butchers sold meat from diseased animals at cheap prices; cows' milk was adulterated with water and chalk; butter was adulterated with copper in order to improve its colour. The widespread adulteration of food in the first part of the nineteenth century meant that many people suffered from diarrhoea and food poisoning.

Water

The rapid expansion of Britain's towns and cities in the early nineteenth century placed water supplies under severe pressure. In working-class districts it was very rare for anyone to have piped water in their home. Water companies supplied water to pumps in the streets and courts. In poorer areas, it was common for whole streets to share a single pump. Often, landlords paid only a small sum to the water companies for the most basic provision. Water might then be available for only two or three hours a day.

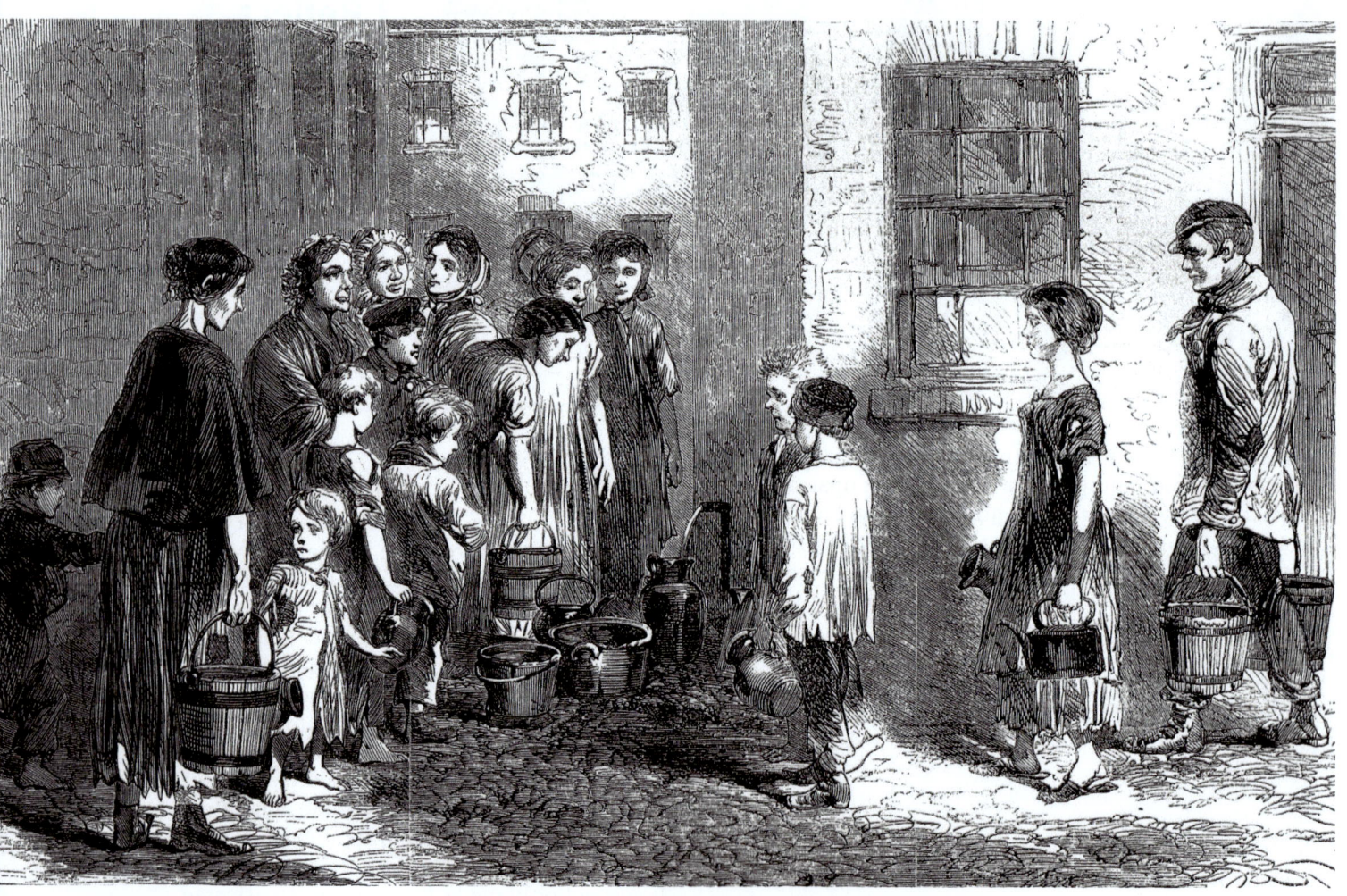

▲ An engraving of people queuing for water. The *Illustrated News*, 1864

Reflect

What can this engraving tell us about the difficulties of obtaining water in the mid-nineteenth century?

Poor families were sometimes unable to afford the water company's charges, and, in some places, a water company did not exist at all. In these situations, people obtained water from the town's river, or they might have to walk a long distance to collect water from a spring, stream or pond. No wonder some people preferred to collect rainwater in cisterns or butts like the ones on Doré's engraving of London on page 57.

All water supplies in the early nineteenth century were dirty. Water companies frequently pumped water from polluted rivers. Springs, streams and ponds were often impure. Rainwater which had fallen through the smoke-filled sky could be unfit to drink. Middle-class families filtered their drinking water, but this was not an option for poor families. In the summer months, when the water was at its dirtiest, typhoid took many lives in the poorest districts. No one was aware that the disease was caused by germs in their dirty drinking water.

Why were there such huge changes in the people's health, 1750–1900?

Waste

The biggest health problem in the first part of the nineteenth century was the disposal of human waste. The existing sewers in towns had been built to drain the streets of rainwater, not to carry away human excrement. Newly built areas of working-class housing rarely had sewers. As a result, pools of stinking water often filled the streets and courts. In the first half of the nineteenth century, people continued to use privies as they had done for hundreds of years. People living in through houses sometimes had their own privy in the back yard, but many families in back-to-back houses shared privies with their neighbours. In some places, more than ten houses might have shared a single privy.

The sewage from 'midden privies' simply collected in a large hole underneath. Some privies were connected to a cesspool – a brick container usually about six feet deep and four feet wide. When cesspools were full they were emptied by 'night soil men' who scooped out the sewage with a bucket, loaded it onto a cart and sold it to local farmers. When landlords did not pay for night soil men, the cesspools overflowed into the yards and courts. Some cesspools were water-tight, but others were designed to leak so that liquid could seep out into the surrounding soil, leaving a more solid sludge for the night soil men to collect.

If a leaking cesspool or midden was close to a well or a pump which supplied people with drinking water, it could be fatal. People in the early nineteenth century thought that the 'miasma' from middens and cesspools was unhealthy, but nobody understood that the real danger came from germs in infected water.

People had used privies, cesspools and night soil men for hundreds of years, but the growing urban population of industrial Britain placed this system of sewage removal under severe pressure. The situation reached crisis point in the early nineteenth century because more middle and upper class people started to use water closets (flushing toilets). At first, water closets were connected to cesspools but, between 1800 and 1830, they were linked to the sewers. In many towns and cities, these emptied directly into the rivers from which the water companies obtained their water. Many people, even the middle classes, now received diluted excrement for drinking, cooking and washing – and paid for it!

Reflect

What point was the cartoonist making in the image below? How did the cartoonist do this so effectively?

▼ 'Dirty Father Thames', a cartoon from *Punch* magazine, 7 October 1848

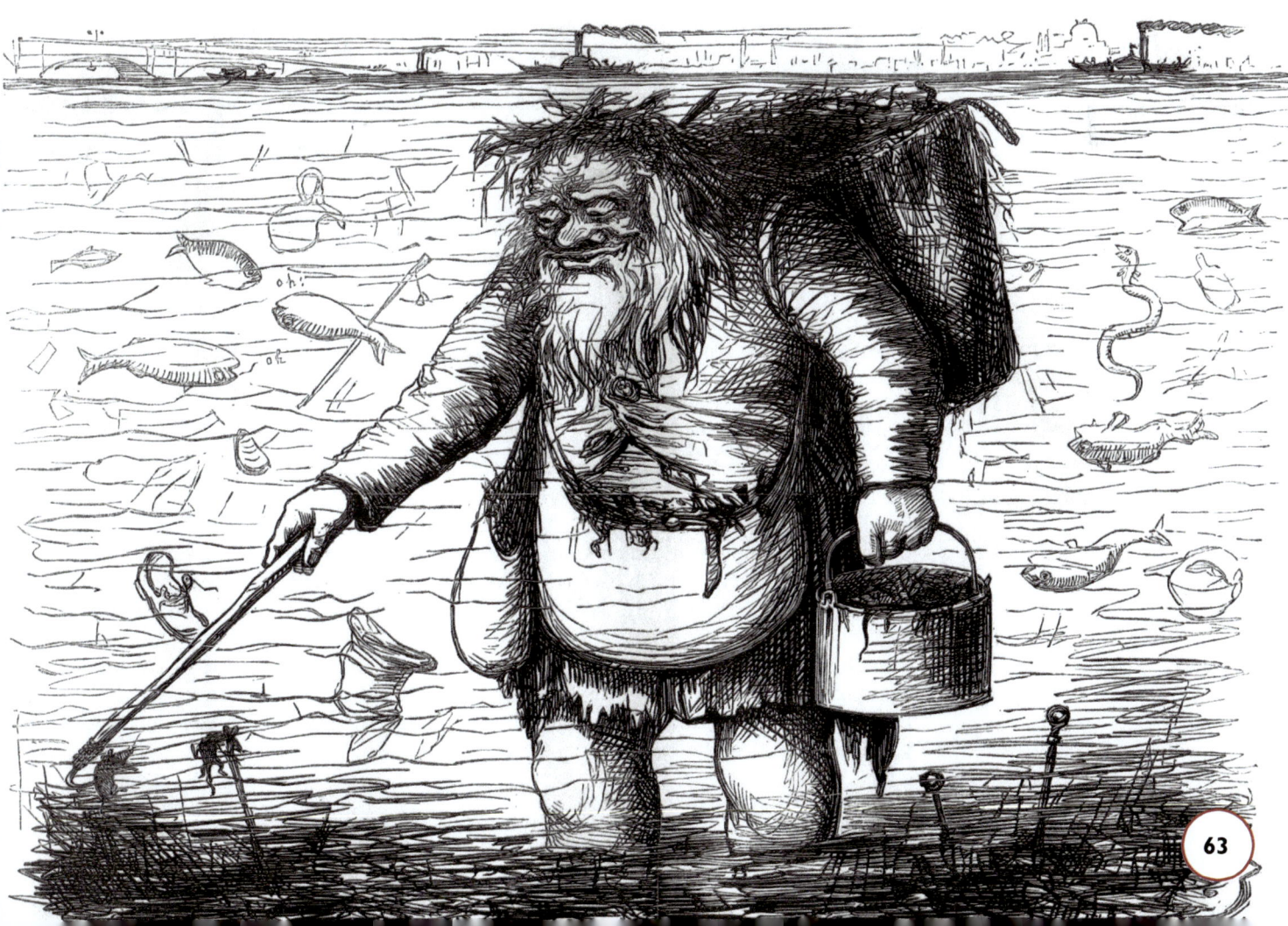

Disease and death: responses to cholera

Many of the diseases which shortened people's lives in the period 1750–1900 had been present in Britain during the medieval and early modern periods. However, the overcrowding, poor diet and terrible sanitation which people experienced in towns and cities made them even bigger killers in the early industrial period.

> ## Record
> Make a table like this one listing the five diseases described below. Explain how each disease was linked to aspects of people's living conditions in early industrial Britain, for example, overcrowding, damp houses, poor diet, poor sanitation.
>
> | Disease | Link to living conditions |
> |---------|---------------------------|
> | | |

Five common diseases in early industrial Britain

Tuberculosis (also called consumption or TB). This was the largest killer in the nineteenth century. The disease was spread from person to person in the droplets of water produced when coughing. It thrived in overcrowded and poorly ventilated houses. TB was sometimes spread through unpasteurised cows' milk too. The disease attacked the lungs and caused people to spit up blood.

Influenza. The virus was transmitted through coughing and sneezing. It caused fever, shivering, severe headaches and vomiting. There were regular flu outbreaks throughout the nineteenth century.

Diphtheria. This was another disease spread through coughing and sneezing. It was also transmitted through contact with the clothing of an infected person. Diphtheria particularly affected children, causing swollen glands, fever and severe headaches.

Typhoid (also called enteric fever). A disease spread through food or water contaminated with human waste. It was sometimes carried by flies which infected food. Prince Albert, Queen Victoria's husband, died of typhoid fever in 1861 at the age of 42. The disease caused fever, severe headaches and diarrhoea.

Typhus. The disease was sometimes confused with typhoid because it had similar symptoms. The virus was transmitted by bites from body lice. It therefore thrived in neighbourhoods where there was overcrowding and where people struggled to keep their clothes and bodies clean.

These five diseases, together with other killers such as bronchitis, pneumonia, smallpox, whooping cough, measles and scarlet fever, had a terrible impact on people's life expectancy in the early nineteenth century. In 1841 average life expectancy at birth was 26.6 years in Manchester, 28.1 years in Liverpool and 27 years in Glasgow. Within individual cities, people's chances of a premature death depended on who they were and where they lived. In Ancoats, the poorest part of Manchester, where disease took the lives of many babies and infants, the average age of death was just fourteen. This shockingly low life expectancy in industrial Britain was partly caused by a new and terrifying disease which reached Britain in October 1831 – cholera.

Why were there such huge changes in the people's health, 1750–1900?

Cholera in Leeds

On Thursday 5 April 1832, a small news item in a Leeds newspaper filled its readers with fear. Cholera had broken out in the canal port of Goole, just forty miles away from Leeds. The epidemic had begun in India, entering Britain through the north eastern port of Sunderland in October 1831. In the following months, it spread across much of the country. Cholera was a terrifying disease. It killed quickly and nastily. Infected people immediately suffered violent vomiting and stomach cramps. A terrible diarrhoea caused them to produce a yellowish watery liquid. The body dehydrated, the pulse weakened and the skin turned blue. Victims were often dead within one or two days.

Cholera reached Leeds on 28 May 1832. The first to die was the two-year-old son of an Irish woollen weaver. The family lived in Blue Bell Fold, a cramped and dirty yard in one of the poorer parts of the city. The houses were built next to a stinking stream which flowed into the River Aire. The disease spread quickly. Within a few days, several people in Blue Bell Fold had died. Cholera soon began to radiate outwards across Leeds. By the end of July, there had been 427 cases and 187 people had died. Most of the victims lived in overcrowded yards which contained some of the worst housing in Leeds. In Boot and Shoe Yard, for example, around ten people shared each of the small back-to-back houses. There was no water within a quarter of a mile, and only three privies for the 340 people in the yard.

▼ A photograph of a Leeds yard, 1901

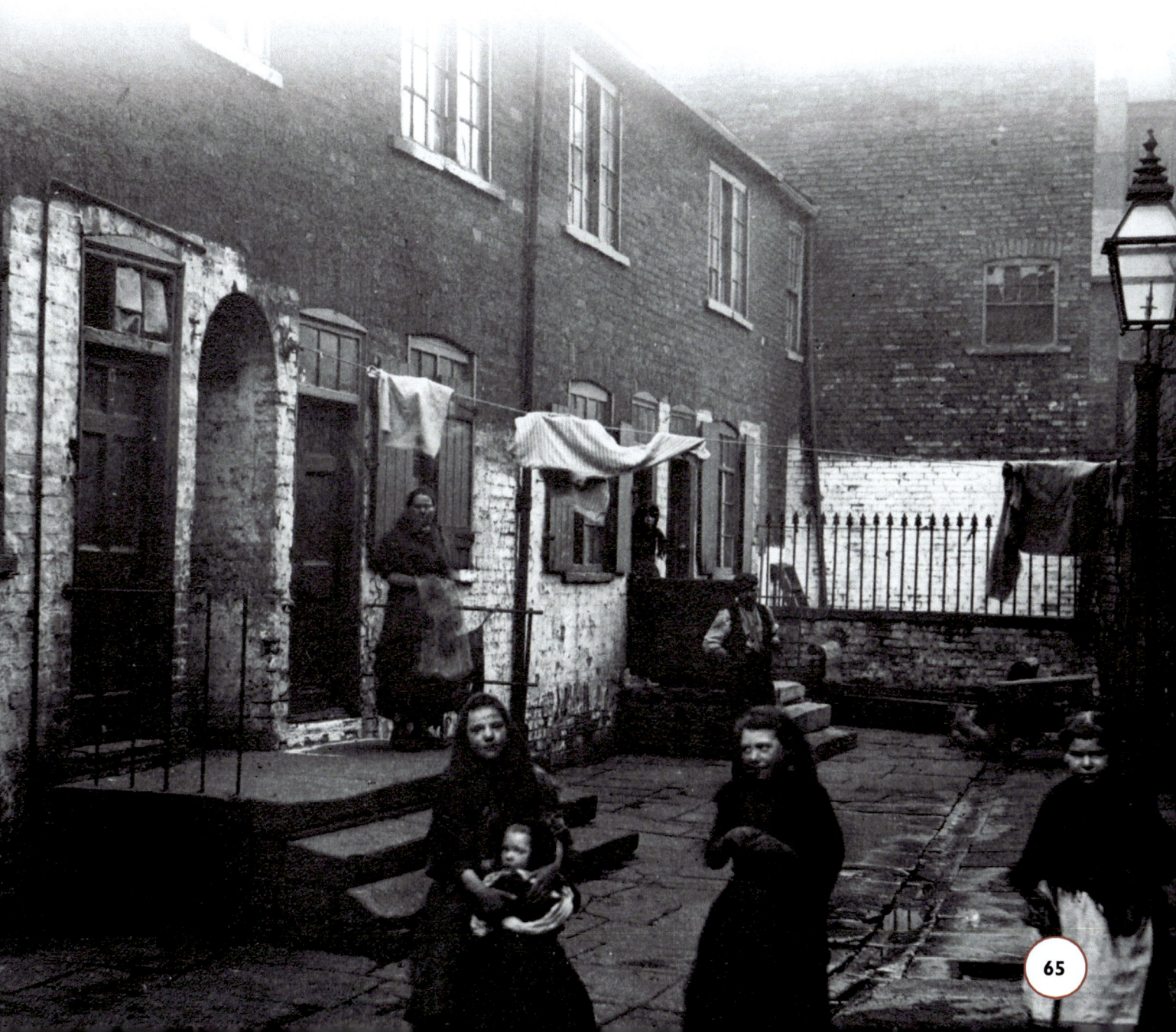

Many of the details of the Leeds cholera outbreak are found in the 1833 report published by Dr Robert Baker, a surgeon who worked for the Leeds Board of Health. Baker's report clearly revealed the link between dirty living conditions and the spread of cholera in Leeds. He carefully recorded each case of cholera and produced a map using dark shading to show the dirtiest parts of the town. Baker was convinced that the bad air produced by dirty streams, overflowing cesspits and dunghills caused the spread of cholera. We now know that this miasma theory was incorrect. Cholera was spread when people drank water contaminated by the excrement of victims. However, Baker did provide evidence of the connection between dirt and disease. His emphasis on the need to clean up areas of dirty housing was the right one – but for the wrong reasons.

Cholera deaths

Despite Dr Baker's efforts, the cholera epidemic in Leeds raged through the summer of 1832, reaching its peak in August. On 21 August, nineteen people were buried in just one of Leeds's churchyards. There was no known cure for the disease. In desperation, people tried a range of useless remedies such as warm drinks and mustard poultices. As early as June, the Leeds Board of Health began to publish advice on preventing the spread of the disease in the local newspapers and on posters. The Board advised people to wash their whole bodies with soap and water at least once a week, to whitewash the insides of their houses and to open their windows. It strongly advised people to avoid alcohol. In fact, beer would have been much safer to drink than the infected water. The measures introduced by the Leeds Board of Health could not prevent the spread of cholera. Two thirds of the people in Leeds had never been to a church service, but many turned to God as the disease took hold of the city.

As more and more people died of cholera, rumours began to circulate in Leeds that the epidemic was the result of a plot between the doctors and the wealthier classes to do away with people living in poverty. The rumours increased when the Board of Health attempted to quarantine victims in a cholera hospital. People were afraid to allow their loved ones to enter the hospital. On 9 June, an angry crowd surrounded the cholera hospital, shouting threats and breaking windows. Some people in Leeds suggested that the crowd was encouraged by mill owners who felt that quarantining people in hospital would affect their businesses. Cholera riots like the ones in Leeds occurred in several towns and cities across Britain in 1832.

By the end of 1832, 702 people in Leeds had died of cholera. Across Britain, the disease killed around 32,000 people. When the epidemic was over, life in Leeds and the rest of Britain continued much as before. Throughout the 1830s and 1840s Britain's public health crisis deepened. But the first cholera epidemic had shocked the authorities, and the work of Robert Baker had begun to reveal the danger which dirty living conditions held for the people's health.

▼ Robert Baker's Sanitary Map of Leeds, 1842

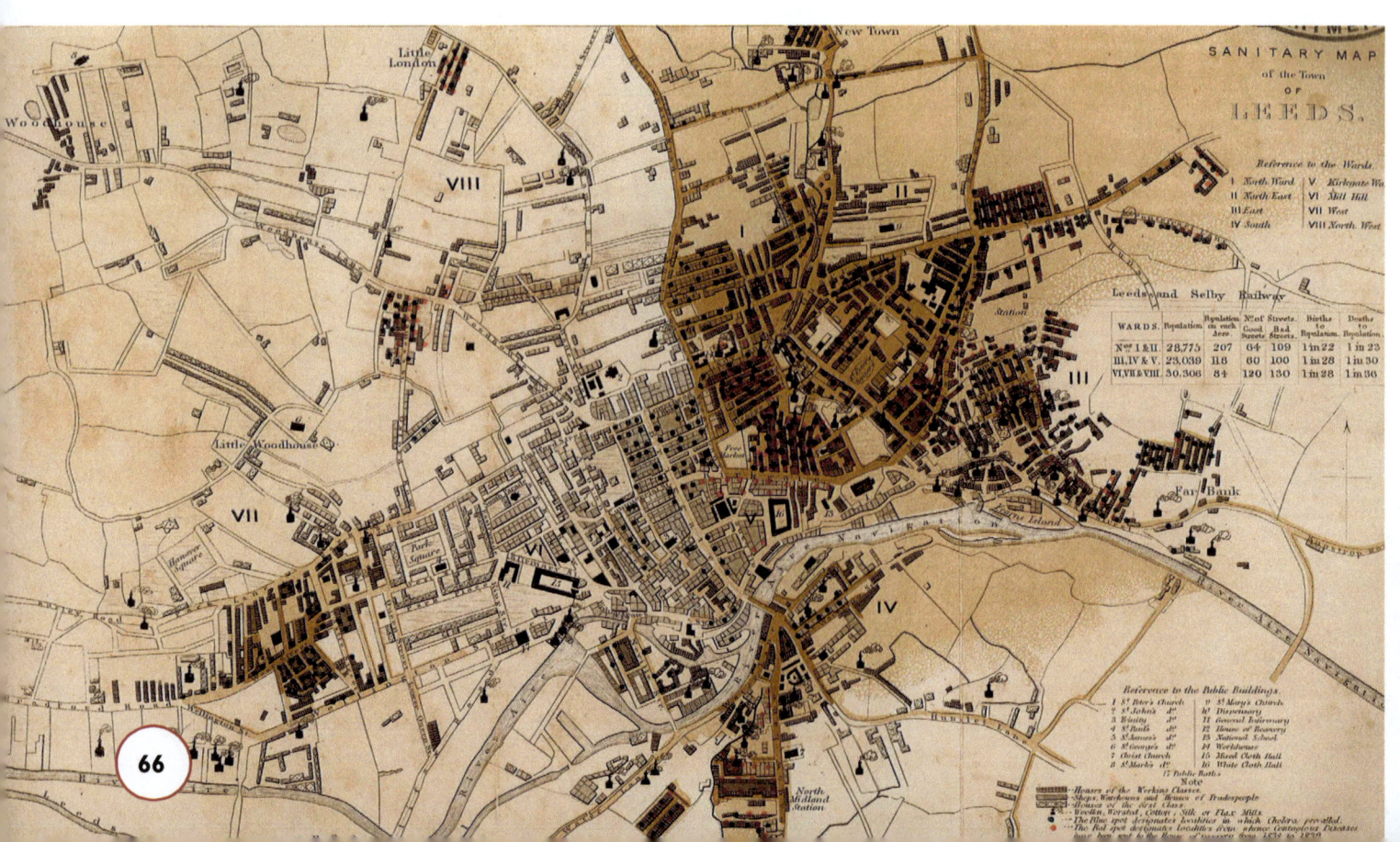

Why were there such huge changes in the people's health, 1750–1900?

Beliefs and responses

We now know that the reason why cholera spread so quickly was because it is a disease transmitted by contaminated water. People become infected by the cholera germ when they drink water contaminated by the excrement of other people already suffering from the disease. That is what made the dirty privies, leaking cesspools and poor water supply of early industrial Britain so dangerous. It was not until the 1850s that cholera was identified as a water-borne disease. In 1832, people had different ideas about what caused the spread of cholera:

- Many people still believed that unexplained events such as disease were the work of God. Some vicars preached that cholera was sent as a punishment for people's sins.
- Some doctors believed that cholera was contagious. They thought that when sick people came into contact with the healthy, the disease was transmitted by touch.
- The most common belief was the miasma theory. This was the theory that the disease was caused by breathing in the bad air (miasma) created by decaying rubbish and human waste.

Reflect

How different were these ideas from people's beliefs about the causes of the Black Death and early modern plague?

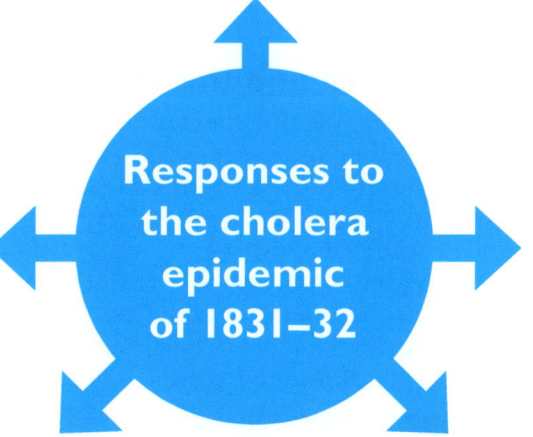

Some boards of health tried to get rid of bad air by burning barrels of tar in the streets. Others paid for people to remove rotting rubbish and dunghills from the streets and courts. In some towns chloride of lime was added to the sewers to make them smell better.

Some local authorities imposed a quarantine. They posted constables on the outskirts of the town to turn away poor people trying to enter. Many towns set up a cholera hospital where victims could be isolated. Some created separate cholera burial grounds.

Responses to the cholera epidemic of 1831–32

Towns were encouraged (but not forced) to set up local boards of health. These volunteer groups relied on donations from individuals and charities. They employed inspectors to monitor outbreaks of cholera and printed posters advising people what to do to prevent the spread of the disease.

In November 1832, the government set up the Central Board of Health. It included two doctors who had been sent to St Petersburg to study the progress of the disease in Russia.

The government sought God's help with a national day of fasting, humiliation and prayer on 2 March 1832.

Record

Produce a summary chart to compare the responses to cholera in 1831–32 with responses to the Black Death in 1348–49 and plague in the sixteenth and seventeenth centuries.

The fight against filth, 1830s–1900

Record

Following the first cholera epidemic of 1831–32 it became obvious that something would have to be done about the filthy living conditions in Britain's towns and cities. From 1840 to 1900, campaigns to reform public health resulted in huge improvements. As you find out about these over the next six pages, complete a 'Fight against filth' chart like the one below to summarise the contributions of different individuals and other factors.

The fight against filth, 1830s–1900		
	Individuals	Other factors
1. Edwin Chadwick and the 1848 Public Health Act		
2. Further changes, 1854–1875		
3. Dirt defeated, 1876–1900		

Edwin Chadwick and the 1848 Public Health Act

Robert Baker was not the only person to connect disease to dirty living conditions. In the 1830s, other doctors, such as James Kay in Manchester and Southwood Smith in London, also wrote reports linking ill-health to poor environments. More evidence was provided by the new statistical societies which published studies of disease and death rates in different parts of Britain. Knowledge about the health of towns also increased after the government introduced the civil registration of births and deaths in 1837. William Farr, the first Registrar-General, required all doctors to state the cause of death on death certificates. This provided more precise knowledge about the impact of different diseases.

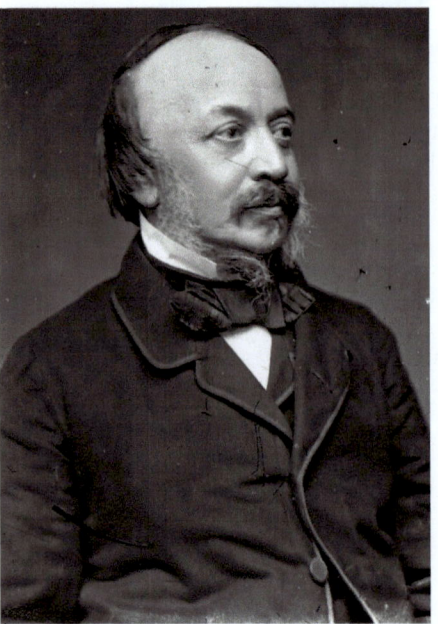

▶ A photograph of Edwin Chadwick, 1850

There is one individual who has been remembered above all others in the campaign for improvements in public health during the 1830s and 1840s. His name was Edwin Chadwick.

Edwin Chadwick's interest in public health grew directly from his work with the Poor Law Commission. Chadwick became convinced that the main cause of poverty was ill health, and that this was the result of people's filthy living conditions. In the late 1830s, Chadwick led a major investigation into the people's health. His famous *Report on the Sanitary Condition of the Labouring Population of Britain* was published in 1842. This massive report was based on detailed evidence provided by doctors and officials from all over the country. It contained shocking details of the public health crisis and sold more copies than any previous government report.

Reflect

How were other factors, as well as individuals, responsible for changing attitudes to public health in the 1830s?

Why were there such huge changes in the people's health, 1750–1900?

Chadwick's *Sanitary Report* of 1842 provided a clear solution to the problem of ill health. He proposed that a national public health authority should be set up, and that it should force local boards of health to provide clean water and new sewerage systems. All cesspools should be replaced with water closets connected to sewers. A constant supply of water should be provided for people to use in their homes and to flush the sewers. The old, flat-bottomed sewers should be replaced with glazed, egg-shaped sewers, flushed by water pressure. Liquid sewage should be recycled into fertiliser on sewage farms. All this should be paid for by an increase in the rates collected from middle-class property owners.

There was a lot of opposition to Chadwick's proposals. Many people thought that it was not the job of central government to interfere in the lives of people in individual towns and cities. The water companies did not want things to change in case it affected their profits. Property owners objected to the suggestion of an increase in rates. However, the pressure for change grew when other voices were added to Chadwick's during the 1840s. In 1844 the Health of Towns Association was formed. It was supported by many leading politicians and Church leaders, and added weight to Chadwick's arguments. By the late 1840s, the pressure for public health reform was unstoppable. In 1848, just as Britain faced the threat of another cholera epidemic, the government passed the Public Health Act. This was the first major law in Britain dealing with public health.

The 1848 Public Health Act was an important step forward in improving the people's health. The belief in *laissez-faire* seemed to be weakening as more people accepted that the government had a role to play in improving people's health. Overall, however, the Act had limited impact. The 1848 Public Health Act was *permissive* rather than *compulsory* – it *allowed* local authorities to clean up their towns, but did not *force* them to take action unless the death rate was high. By the end of 1853, only 163 places had set up a local board of health. There was still plenty of room for improvement in the people's health.

▼ A cartoon titled 'A Court for King Cholera', 1852

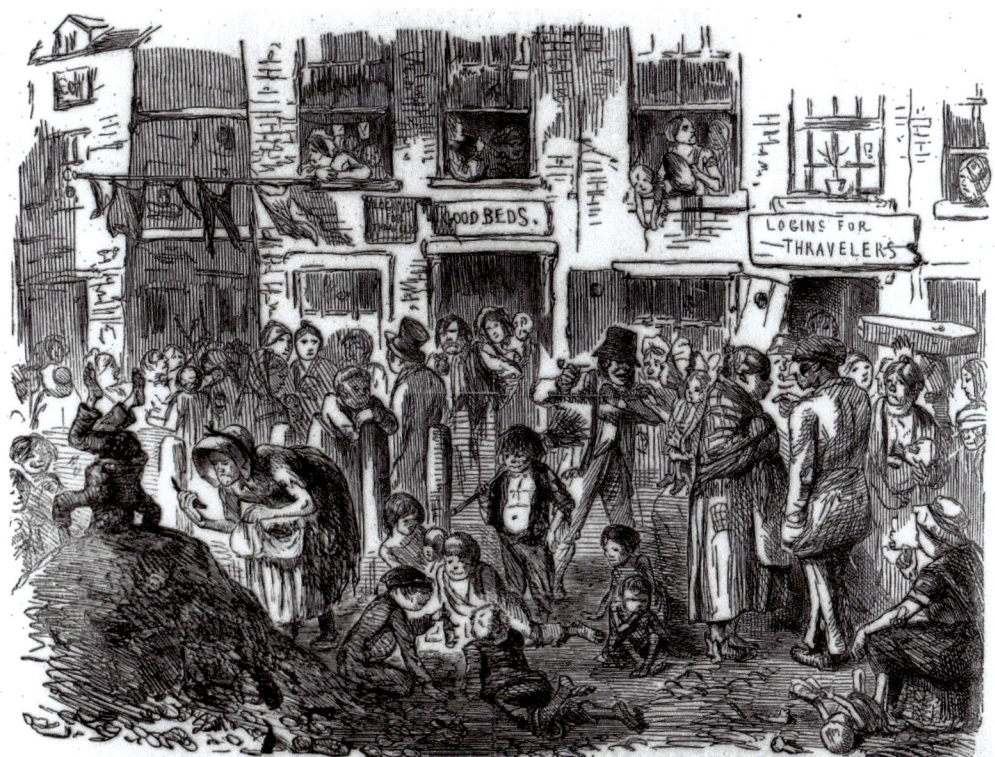

Public Health Act 1848

- Set up the General Board of Health which was given powers until 1854. Chadwick became one of the commissioners.
- Allowed a local board to be set up if ten per cent of ratepayers wanted one.
- Forced towns to set up a board of health where the death rate was higher than 23 per 1,000.
- Allowed boards of health to connect houses to sewers, to make sure that houses had a clean water supply and to set rates to pay for improvements.
- Did not apply to Scotland or to London.

Reflect

1. What made the 1848 Public Health Act a big step forward?
2. What were the limitations of the Act?

Reflect

In this cartoon the cartoonist drew attention to the filthy living conditions in London. How did the cartoonist do this?

Further changes, 1854–1875

> ### Record
> In the two decades after 1854 there were forces at work which led to further changes in the people's health. As you find out about the individuals and other factors involved, remember to add points to the two columns in your 'Fight against filth' chart. Use a different colour to add any factors which you think were still holding back improvements in public health in the period 1854–1875.

1854: John Snow linked cholera to infected water

John Snow was a London doctor who became convinced that cholera was carried in water. When cholera struck Britain again in 1854, Snow made a scientific study of the cholera victims near his surgery in Soho. He discovered that some victims were using the same pump in Broad Street. After Snow gained permission to remove the handle of the pump there were no more cases of cholera in the area. John Snow's published study demonstrated that cholera was a water-borne disease, but many people, including Chadwick, continued to support the miasma theory.

1854: The cholera germ identified

Filippo Pacini was an Italian doctor working in Florence. During the 1854 cholera epidemic he performed autopsies on cholera victims and examined samples from their intestines under his microscope. Pacini discovered the comma-shaped organism which caused cholera and published a scientific paper to explain his discovery. His work was completely overlooked. John Snow knew nothing of Pacini's work in far-away Italy.

1855: The work of John Simon

John Simon was a leading London surgeon who was appointed as Medical Officer to the General Board of Health in 1855. Over the next twenty years he carried out a number precise scientific enquiries into the links between living conditions and disease. Simon's reports were important in persuading the government to intervene in public health.

1858: 'The Great Stink'

In the scorching summer of 1858 the River Thames dried up so much that the smell of sewage from the river became unbearable. To kill the smell, the windows in the House of Commons were draped with curtains soaked in chloride of lime, but it was still impossible for MPs to continue with their debates. The MPs decided that something had to be done about London's sewage problem. They turned to the chief engineer of the Metropolitan Board of Works, Joseph Bazalgette. Between 1858 and 1865, Bazalgette built 1300 miles of sewers across London. It was a remarkable achievement. (You will find out more about Bazalgette's sewers in the Closer Look on pages 74–75.)

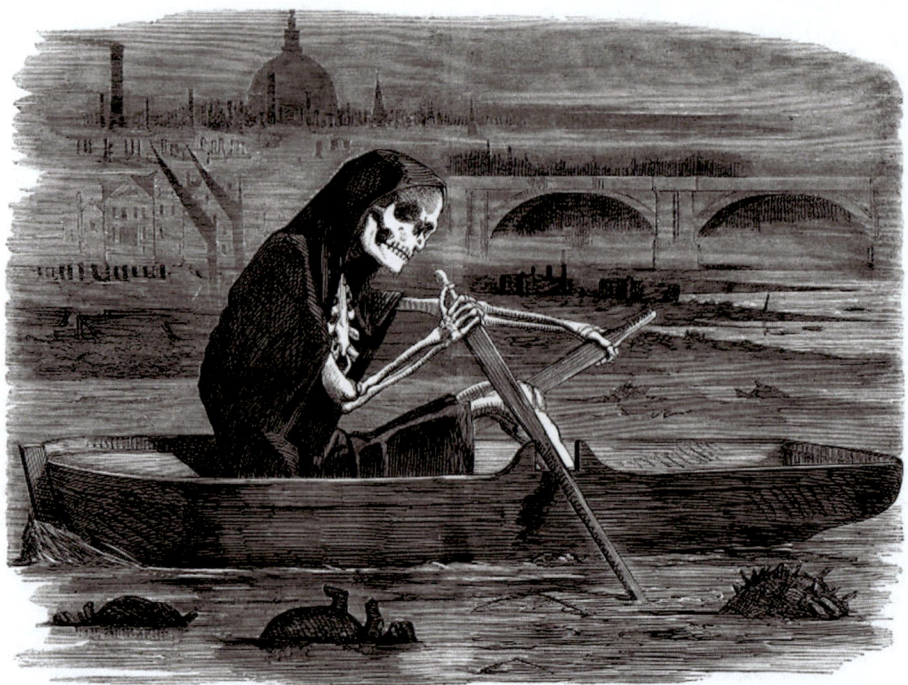

◂ A cartoon titled 'The Silent Highwayman', from *Punch* magazine, 1858

> ### Reflect
> What is the message of this cartoon?

Why were there such huge changes in the people's health, 1750–1900?

1860: The Pure Food Act
This was the first law in Britain that tried to prevent the adulteration of food. In 1872, a stronger law was passed giving more powers to inspectors.

1861: Pasteur's germ theory
In France, the scientist Louis Pasteur published the germ theory following his research into contaminated wine (see page 58). This explained the results which John Snow had recorded. However, many doctors continued to believe in the miasma theory. The germ theory of disease was not widely accepted until the 1880s.

1866: Another cholera epidemic
This outbreak of cholera was less severe than in 1832, 1848 and 1854. In London, the lower number of deaths was mainly due to Bazalgette's sewers. However, politicians were outraged when 7,000 people died because the London Water Company accidentally allowed sewage from a district where cholera was raging to pollute the water supply of people in the East End of London.

1867: Working-class men got the vote
In 1867, Parliament passed a Reform Act which gave working-class men in towns and cities the right to vote for MPs and for town councillors. Now, politicians had to listen to people living in poverty who could vote them out of power.

1867: Pail privies
Pail privies, first used by the corporation in Rochdale, were much better for public health than midden privies. Underneath each privy seat was a pail (bucket) which could be emptied regularly by the local authority. In 1867, the new Medical Officer of Health in Manchester, John Lee, began to replace the city's midden privies with pail privies. By the end of the nineteenth century, pail privies were used in many towns across Britain.

1872: Benjamin Disraeli promised change
Benjamin Disraeli, the leader of the Conservative Party, was determined to win the support of the new working-class voters. In 1872, he made a speech in Manchester promising that he would provide 'pure air, pure water and the inspection of unhealthy houses'. When Disraeli became Prime Minister in 1874 his government made public health a priority.

1873: Imported food and growing wealth
The price of food started to drop when cheap imports of grain arrived from America. In the 1870s, the income of most working-class people began to rise. Cheaper food and higher incomes led to a higher standard of living and better health for many families.

1875: The Public Health Act
The government passed a Public Health Act in 1875 which was much stronger than the 1848 Act. The 1875 Act **forced** councils to clean up their towns:

- All local authorities had to appoint a medical officer and a sanitary inspector.
- Local authorities had to take responsibility for sewers, water supplies, rubbish collection, public toilets and public parks.
- All new houses had to have piped water and proper toilets, drains and sewers.
- Sanitary inspectors had to inspect slaughterhouses and shops to prevent the sale of contaminated food.

▼ A pail privy

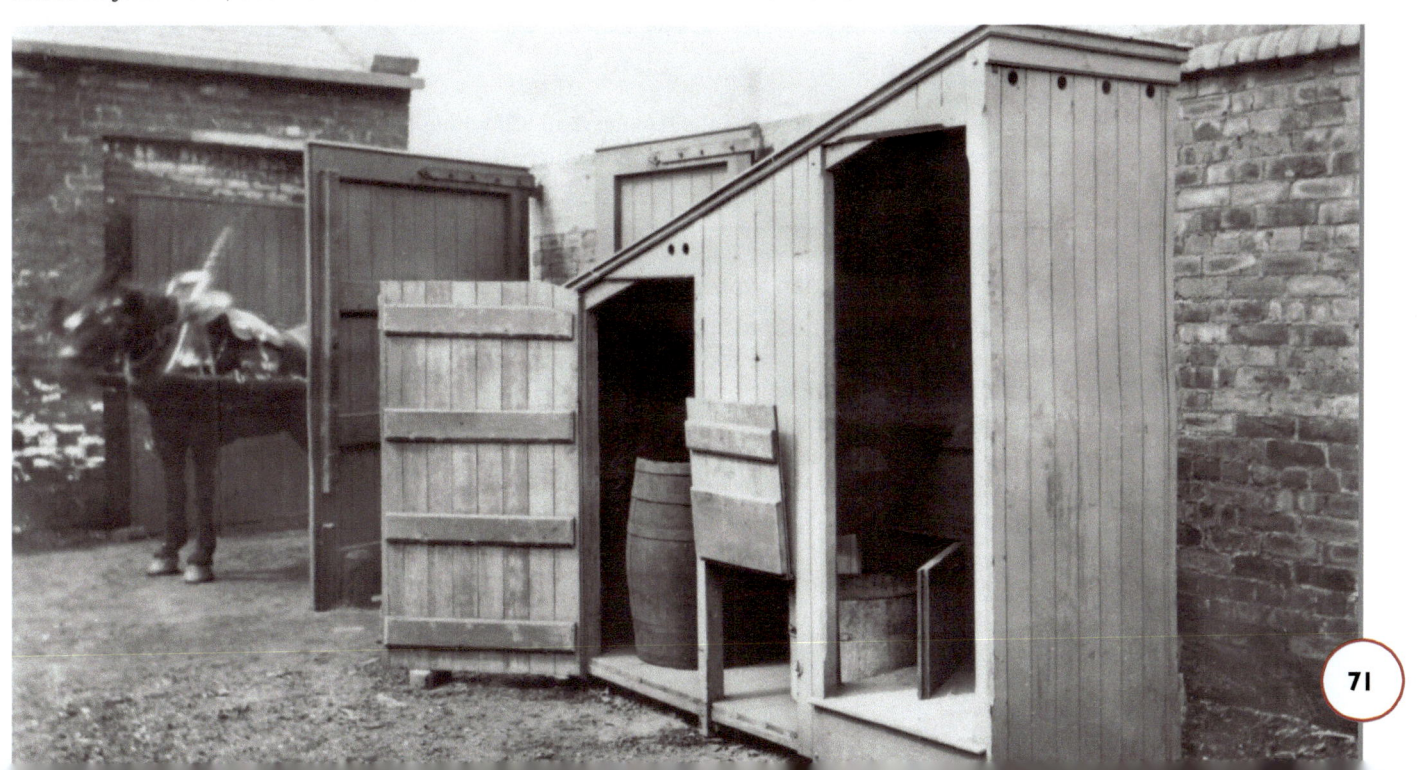

Dirt defeated, 1875–1900

> ### Record
> As you find out about changes after 1875 on the following pages, remember to start a final row in your 'Fight against filth' chart and add points in the two columns.

By 1875, there had been a big shift in people's attitudes towards public health. Industry and trade had made Britain the wealthiest country in the world, and many people believed that some of this wealth should be spent on improving the people's health. The era of *laissez-faire* was over and it was generally accepted that central and local government had a responsibility to protect the health of the people. In the years between 1875 and the end of the century, these beliefs became even stronger, and new political and social forces emerged which would further improve the people's health.

The Women's Co-operative Guild

By the end of the nineteenth century, working-class people were forming political and industrial organisations which demanded change. One of these was the Women's Co-operative Guild which held its first meeting at Hebden Bridge in 1883. The Women's Co-operative Guild campaigned to improve the political and legal status of women. It also fought for government action in health matters such as maternity care for pregnant women, free school meals for poor children, better housing and clean water. Women were becoming a powerful force in the campaign to improve public health.

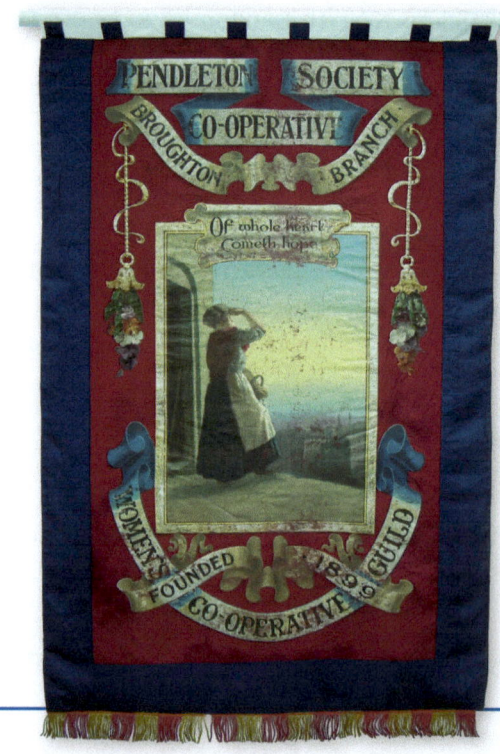

▶ The banner of the Broughton branch of the Women's Co-operative Guild

> ### Reflect
> The words in the centre of the banner read 'Of whole heart cometh hope' and the image shows a woman looking out across an industrial landscape. What can the banner tell us about the aims of the women who belonged to the Guild?

Civic pride and clean water

Towards the end of the nineteenth century, mayors and councillors in many parts of Britain began to spend huge sums of money on building schemes which demonstrated the power and prosperity of their towns and cities. They built magnificent town halls, squares, shopping streets, art galleries, concert halls, libraries and museums. Another expression of this civic pride was the money which some local authorities spent on huge engineering projects to bring clean water to their town or city.

By the late 1870s, Manchester was still without an adequate supply of clean drinking water. Manchester Corporation drew up a plan to dam Thirlmere Lake in the Lake District, raise the level of the lake and construct a 96-mile aqueduct to

Why were there such huge changes in the people's health, 1750–1900?

carry water from the newly-created reservoir into the centre of Manchester. Parliament approved the Thirlmere Water Scheme in 1879. It was a massive engineering project which took 3,000 men eight years to complete. The first water gushed out of the specially-built ceremonial fountain in Albert Square, Manchester, on 13 October 1894. By 1900, water schemes across Britain meant that nearly everyone had a constant supply of clean drinking water piped to their house.

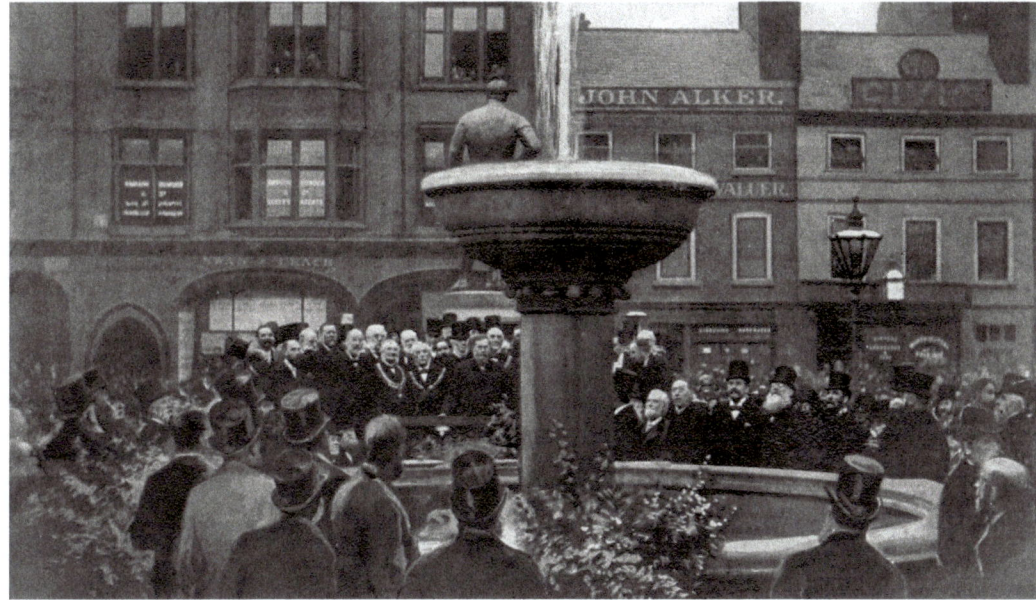

◀ A photograph of the official opening of the Thirlmere Water Scheme in Albert Square, Manchester, 13 October 1894

> **Reflect**
>
> How can you tell that Manchester's civic leaders were proud of their achievement?

Civic pride and new housing

Another expression of civic pride in the late nineteenth century was the construction of local authority housing which provided people with decent homes. In 1885, Manchester Corporation began to demolish some of the worst slums in the city. This photograph shows Victoria Square which was built in Ancoats, one of Manchester's worst slum districts, in 1894. The block contained 235 two-roomed dwellings. There were laundries in the corner turrets and refuse chutes on every floor. Dwellings were arranged in pairs with each pair sharing a sink and a privy.

Manchester and other cities had made a start on improving people's housing, but there was still a long way to go. By 1900, nearly everyone in Britain had clean water, but not decent housing, good food and clean air. These problems, and some totally new threats to the people's health, would be the challenges of the twentieth century.

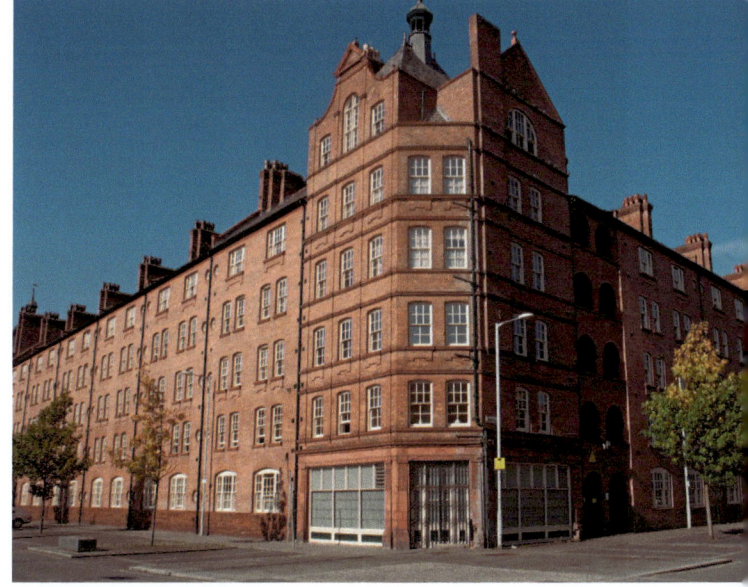

▶ Victoria Square dwellings

> ## Review
>
> Use all the notes you have made on the period 1750–1900 to answer the following question:
>
> 'The work of Edwin Chadwick was the most important factor in improving the health of towns in the nineteenth century.'
>
> How far do you agree with this statement? Give reasons for your answer.

CLOSER LOOK 3

Joseph Bazalgette and the revolution in London's sewers

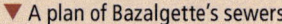

▲ Joseph Bazalgette

This is Joseph Bazalgette. His moustache was a remarkable achievement, but we remember Bazalgette for something even greater – saving the lives of thousands of Londoners. Bazalgette began his career as a railway engineer. In 1855, the Metropolitan Board of Works was founded to improve London's environment and Bazalgette became its chief engineer. The urgent task was to construct a system of sewers which would avoid London's sewage flowing directly into the central part of the River Thames. Everyone knew that this would be very difficult and expensive. For three years nothing was done, then, in the summer of 1858, came the 'Great Stink'. The government ordered the Metropolitan Board of Works to clean up the river. This was Bazalgette's moment.

Bazalgette designed an entirely new sewerage system for London. His plan was to construct 82 miles of main sewers running from west to east across the city. Three main sewers to the north of the river, and two to the south, would cut across the existing rivers which flowed into the Thames. Smaller street sewers would carry sewage from people's houses into the main sewers. London's filth would flow eastwards across the city, to be dumped in the Thames well downstream of the built up area. Pumping stations on each bank of the river, would pump the sewage into huge covered reservoirs. Twice a day the sewage would be released into the river so that it could flow away on the outgoing tide.

▼ A plan of Bazalgette's sewers

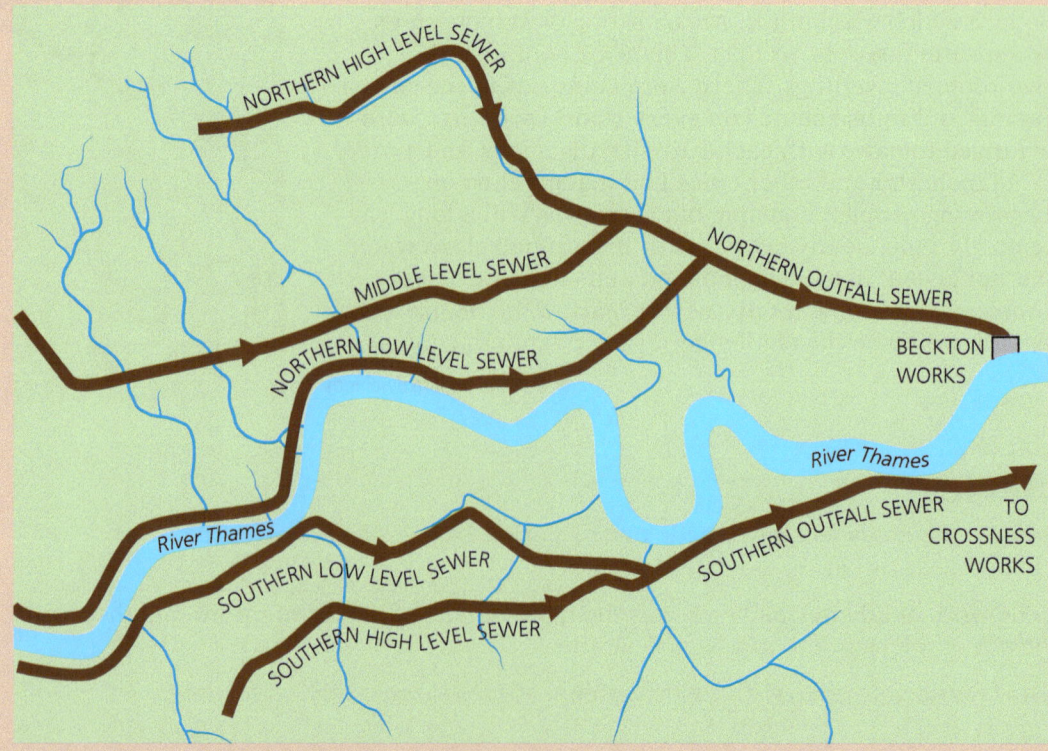

Joseph Bazalgette and the revolution in London's sewers

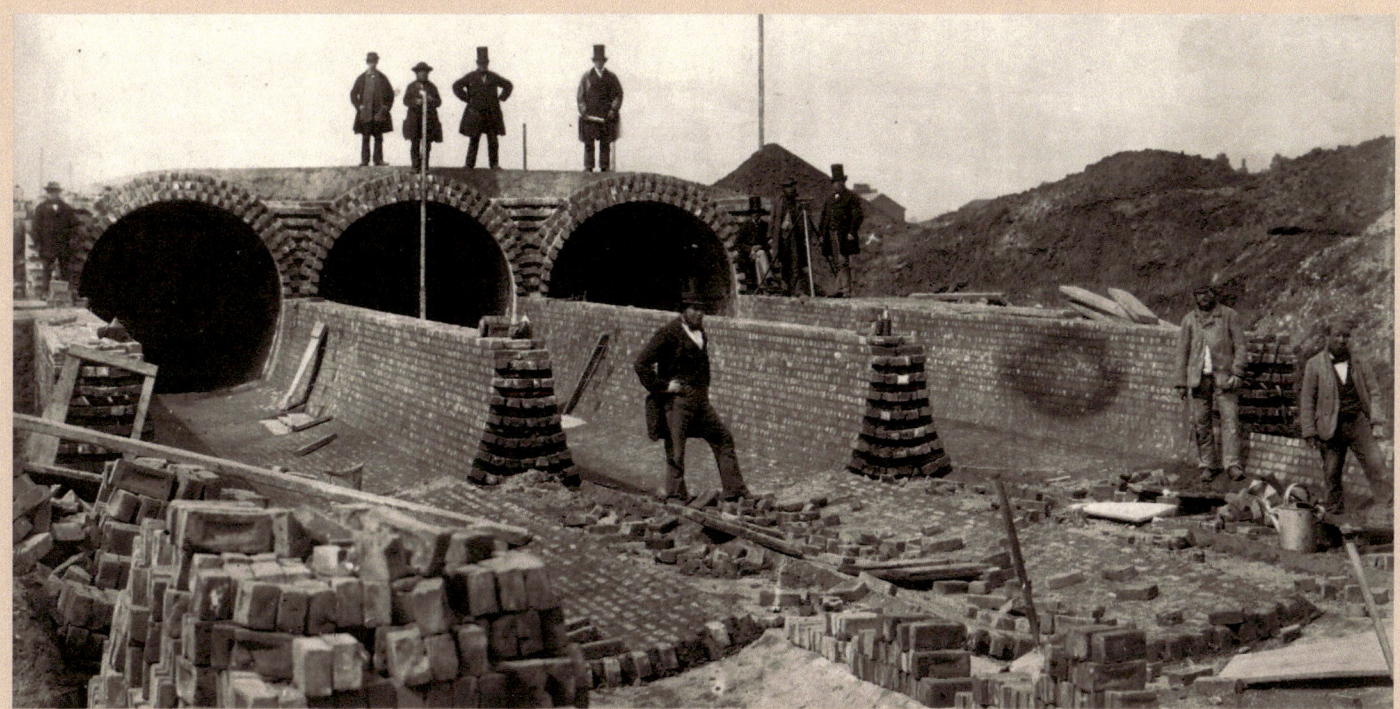

▲ Joseph Bazalgette (top left) viewing the sewers at Abbey Mills Pumping Station on the north bank of the River Thames, 1862

Bazalgette's sewers took seven years to build. Thousands of labourers moved mountains of earth and constructed nearly 1,300 miles of sewers under the streets of what was then the world's largest and busiest city. They used a total of 318 million bricks. Bazalgette was not only a skilled engineer, but also a meticulous and hard-working project manager. He paid careful attention to every detail of the construction and thought very carefully about the exact design of the system. His most brilliant decision was to create enormously wide sewers. Bazalgette calculated how much sewage Londoners produced each day, worked out the diameter of sewer this required, and then doubled it as he knew that London's population density would increase in the future. It is remarkable that his sewers still cope with London's sewage today.

This is a photograph of the interior of Crossness Pumping Station on the south bank of the River Thames. Restoration of this amazing building began in 1985. The four enormous engines in the corners of the building were designed by Bazalgette to pump the sewage into the covered reservoir.

▼ The restored interior of Crossness Pumping Station

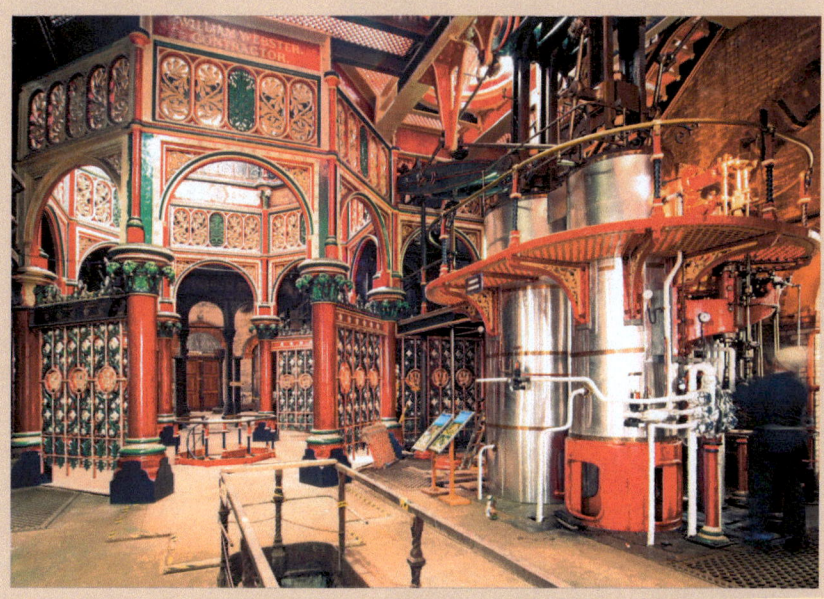

The beautifully painted ironwork makes Crossness look more like a palace than a sewage pumping station. On 4 April 1865, the Prince of Wales came to Crossness to officially open London's new sewer system. Bazalgette made a speech, the Prince turned the wheel which started the four engines, then the 500 guests sat down to lunch in a room next to the engine shed of the sewage pumping station!

Bazalgette's sewers probably made the single biggest contribution to the health of Londoners in the nineteenth century. The belief behind the project – that miasma spread cholera – was wrong, but the new sewerage system prevented the spread of cholera and other water-borne diseases like typhoid. It was a revolution in public health!

4 Better than ever?

Do the changes in public health since 1900 tell a simple story of progress?

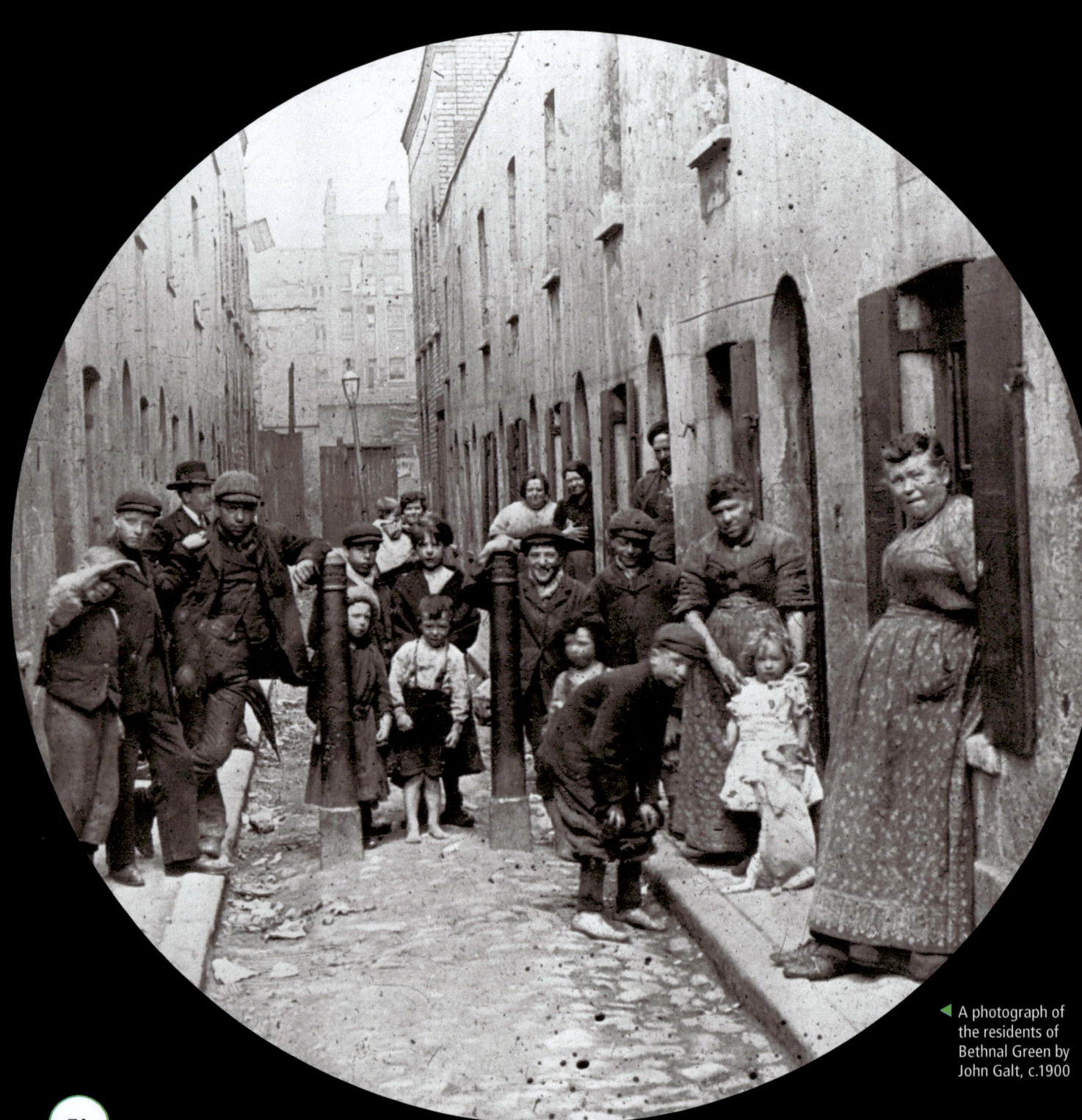

◀ A photograph of the residents of Bethnal Green by John Galt, c.1900

Do the changes in public health since 1900 tell a simple story of progress?

The people looking out at you from this photograph lived in east London around 1900. The picture was taken by John Galt, a Christian missionary and amateur photographer. Galt showed images like this to middle-class audiences at slide shows known as 'magic lantern' shows. He knew that the great improvements in public health care at the end of the nineteenth century had not reached everyone in Britain. He wanted to show the middle classes that for those living in older houses in poorer districts, problems of dirt and disease were as bad as ever.

Galt was not alone. Between 1889 and 1903, Charles Booth, a wealthy merchant with a deep social conscience, published his *Life and Labour of People in London* in several volumes. This showed that 35 per cent of people living in east London were in desperate poverty. The book used new techniques in mapping to show the relative wealth of different parts of the city.

Then, in 1901, Seebohm Rowntree, the son of a famous chocolate manufacturer, published *Poverty: a study of town life* which showed that the city of York was also still plagued by poverty. Families had too little money to live on at the best of times and had no safety net to protect them in old age or when the breadwinner was ill or unemployed. Rowntree used his background as a scientist to gather data of many sorts and proved that the main reason for poverty in York was, quite simply, that wages were too low. This contradicted the views of many Victorians who insisted that people living in poverty brought their problems on themselves by reckless spending or failure to plan ahead.

Despite all the progress made in the previous century, it was clear that Britain still had to tackle some enormous challenges in public health care. But who should be responsible for making changes? Could improvements be made at all and, if so, how? Who would pay the costs? And would all Britain's people feel the benefits this time, or just the rich? Only time would tell.

> **Reflect**
> What signs can you see that Galt, Booth and Rowntree all used modern methods to try to help people living in poverty?

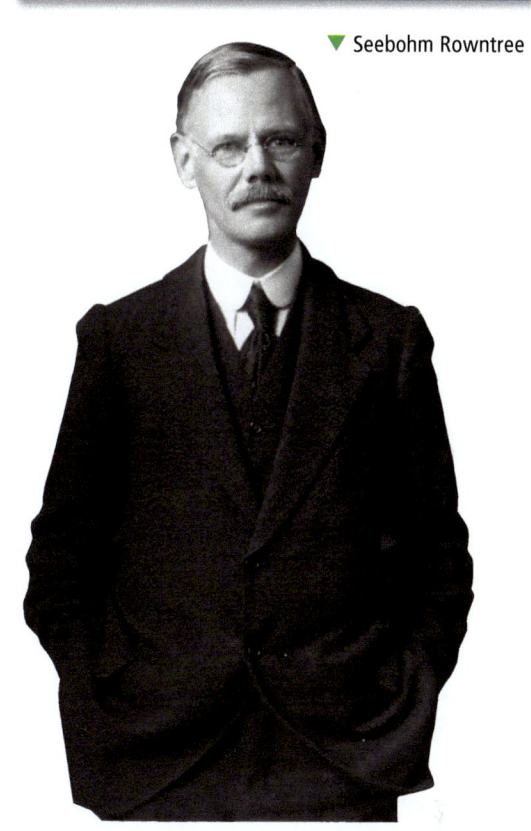

▼ Seebohm Rowntree

The Enquiry

The changes in our public health care since 1900 are so great that you might think that the answer to our enquiry question must be 'Yes – the twentieth century was a simple story of progress in the people's health'. But it is not that easy.

In history, *change* does not always mean progress. It can bring new and even more difficult challenges.

In this enquiry, you will consider each of the following:

1. An overview of the main changes to life in Britain in the twentieth century.
2. How changes in people's living conditions and lifestyles affected their health.
3. How Britain responded to two very different epidemics: the outbreak in 1918 of 'Spanish Influenza' and the spread of AIDS from 1981.
4. How governments have responded to challenges to the British people's health.

At each stage in the enquiry, after the overview, you must track any signs of progress and identify new challenges. Like all historians, you can only reach your judgement about whether there has been progress or not by finding evidence for each side of the argument.

Use a chart for making your notes. It should look like this:

Issue	On the one hand there were signs of progress such as ...	On the other hand there were still significant challenges such as ...
Living conditions		

Britain 1900–2000: an overview

Record
The next four pages summarise different aspects of life in twentieth-century Britain. Read through them quickly and make a list of at least six specific features that you think may have affected people's health at that time. Collect and explain your ideas in a table like this:

Specific feature of life at this time	How I think this may have affected the people's health

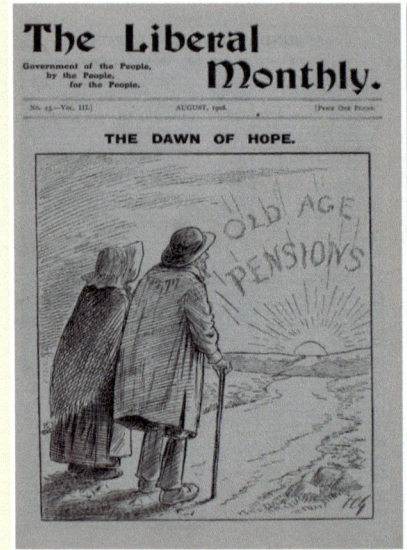

1. Government and welfare c.1900
From the 1880s, most working men over the age of 21 had the right to vote. Governments had to do more to meet the needs of these people if they wanted to gain their support. Between 1906 and 1911, the Liberal Party passed a series of laws to make life more comfortable for people living in poverty. These included the introduction of free school meals and the first state-funded old-age pension. This was the beginning of what we now call the 'Welfare State', where the government uses taxpayers' money to provide for the needs of the whole society, especially the most vulnerable people.

◀ A picture from a Liberal Party pamphlet issued in 1908

2. Science and technology c.1900
Advances in science and technology accelerated around 1900. In 1896, an Act of parliament allowed the first motor cars on British roads, with a speed limit of 14 miles per hour. In the same year, moving picture films were shown for the first time in Britain and cinemas were soon being built. In 1901, the Italian inventor Marconi used enormous kites to lift radio aerials high into the sky and sent a wireless telegraph signal from America to England. These advances in travel and communications meant that people, images and ideas moved around more easily and so changed rapidly over the next century.

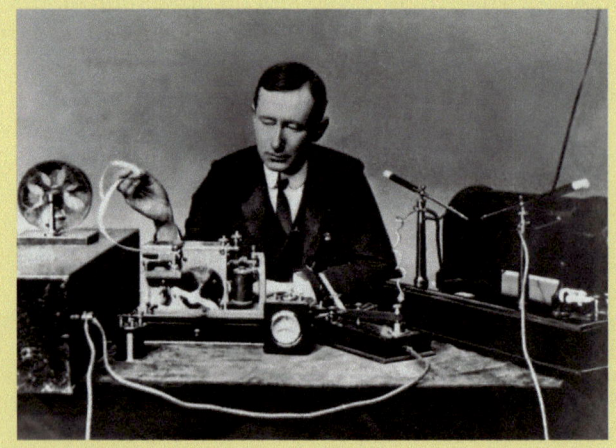

▶ Marconi using his wireless telegraph in 1901

3. Beliefs and values c.1900
In 1900, the majority of people in Britain still attended church and 55 per cent of children went to Sunday school. But, according to some, science showed that God did not exist. They argued that humankind was responsible for its own development. In 1896, the British Humanist Society was founded, insisting that people could lead good lives and improve the world without needing to believe in God. Around the same time, psychiatrists such as Sigmund Freud explained the human mind in ways that challenged what religious people called the 'soul'. The horrors of the First World War of 1914–18 added to the religious doubts of many.

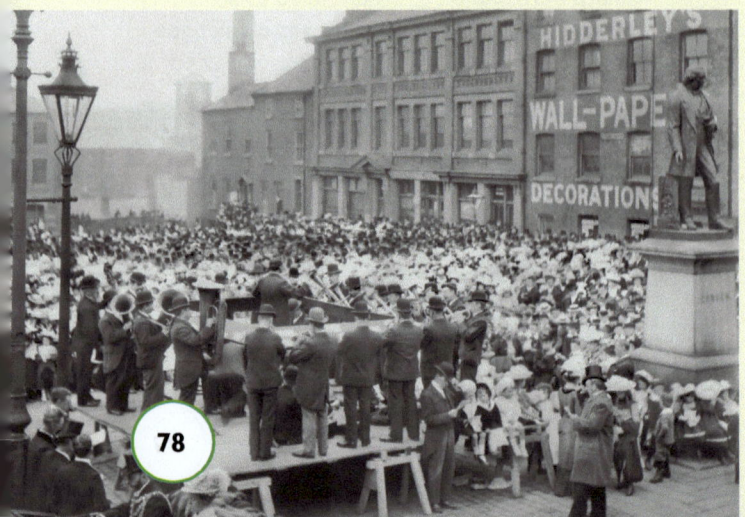

◀ A Sunday school celebration in Stockport, 1896

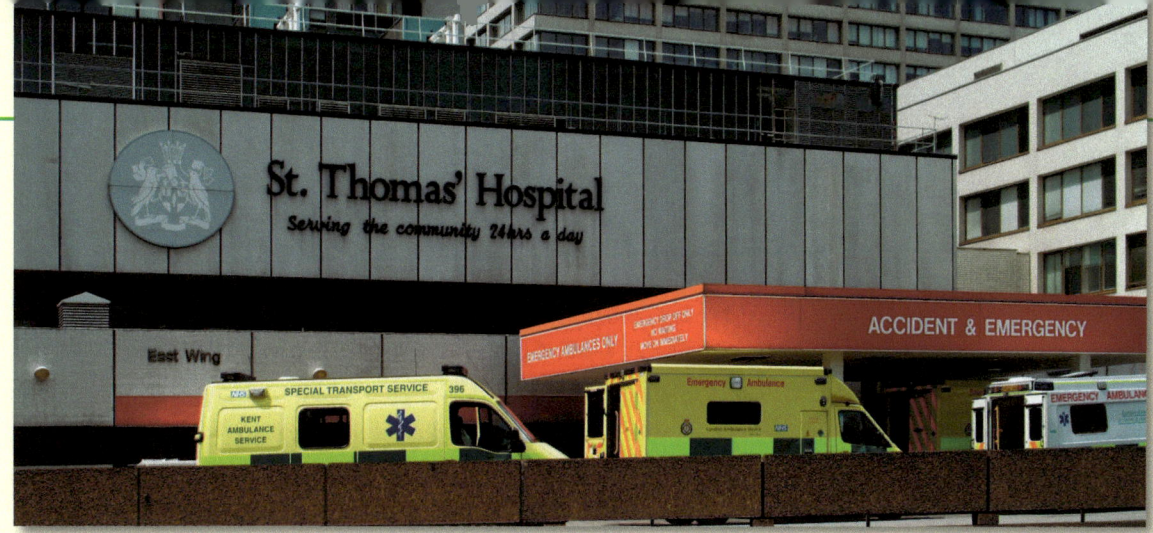

◀ St Thomas' Hospital in London, 2014. This is just one of many hospitals run by the National Health Service using tax payers' money. There were no hospitals like this in 1900

4. Government and welfare c.2000

The Welfare State that started in the 1900s grew throughout the century, especially after many women gained the right to vote in 1918. By 1928, every adult in the country could vote and governments did more and more to provide for their needs. Generally speaking, Labour governments increased spending on the Welfare State while the Conservatives tried to hold down or even cut the costs, but all governments have been far more involved in looking after the British people's needs than was the case before 1900.

The biggest change came at the end of the Second World War. Voters elected a Labour Government that promised to use the power of the state to defeat social problems such as hunger and illness, just as it had been used to defeat Nazi Germany. This led to the creation of the National Health Service in 1948.

By 2010, the costs of the Welfare State and the degree of government control over people's lives had gone too far for many voters. Governments have tried to cut back on its cost while still promising to look after the people.

5. Science and technology c.2000

The world has been transformed by science and technology since 1900. Chemical industries make paints, plastics, weed killers and fertilisers that could not have existed before 1900. The 1960s saw the arrival of the contraceptive pill that did so much to change family planning. Biological sciences have given the world antibiotics, which quickly end many infections that were once fatal, and have opened new understanding of the genes that shape all life. Physics has helped to send humans and machines into space and to create computers and digital communication systems that build and share knowledge at remarkable speed. Cars and aeroplanes now allow people to travel further and more speedily than ever. These developments have often made life easier but they have also been used to make war more deadly and have created new environmental challenges.

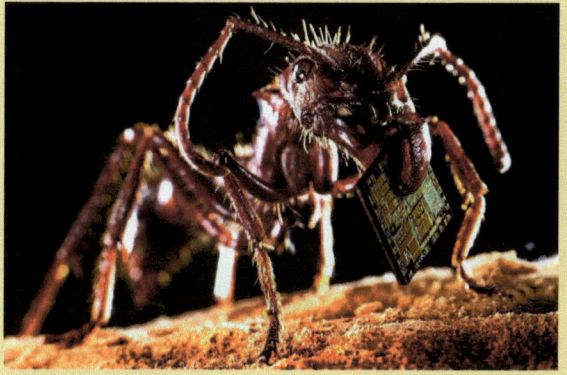

▼ A highly magnified photograph of an ant carrying a microprocessor

6. Beliefs and values c.2000

Another important change came in 1948 when the United Nations Organisation published its Declaration of Human Rights. Since then people have been able to stop governments from ignoring their needs if they can show that they have a right to expect action. This is very different from the centuries when those in power could ignore the mass of society if they wanted to.

In a 2001 survey, over 70 per cent of British people described themselves as Christian but fewer than 10 per cent attended church. Most people in Britain would now probably turn to science rather than prayer to deal with a major social problem.

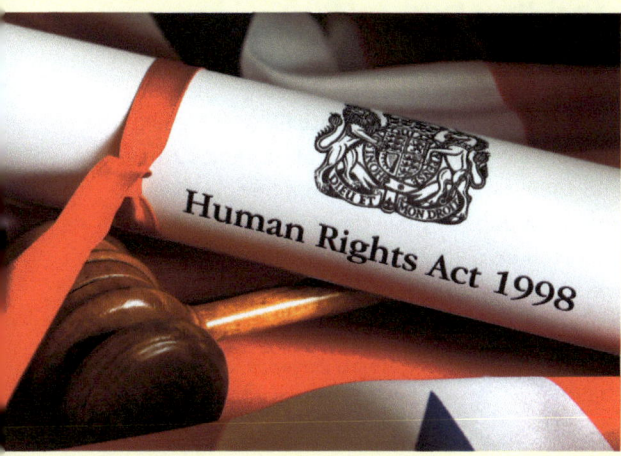

◀ The UK Human Rights Act, 1998

7. Work and wealth c.1900

In 1900, most people in Britain worked with their hands like these coalminers. Some were highly skilled workers while others were just labourers. British factories produced textiles and other goods that were taken in British-made steam ships, powered by British coal and sold to parts of the British Empire all around the world.

The heavy work was mainly done by hand so the workforce was largely made up of men. It was unusual for married women to work. Wives generally stayed at home to look after the house and children. Young women often worked as domestic servants for the middle and upper classes. For the working classes, hours were long and wages were generally low. They usually lived close by each other in poor-quality, rented houses.

Workers tried to improve their conditions through support of the trades unions and the Labour Party that had been formed in 1900. This aimed to make Parliament change laws so that workers' lives would be safer and more comfortable in return for their part in creating Britain's wealth.

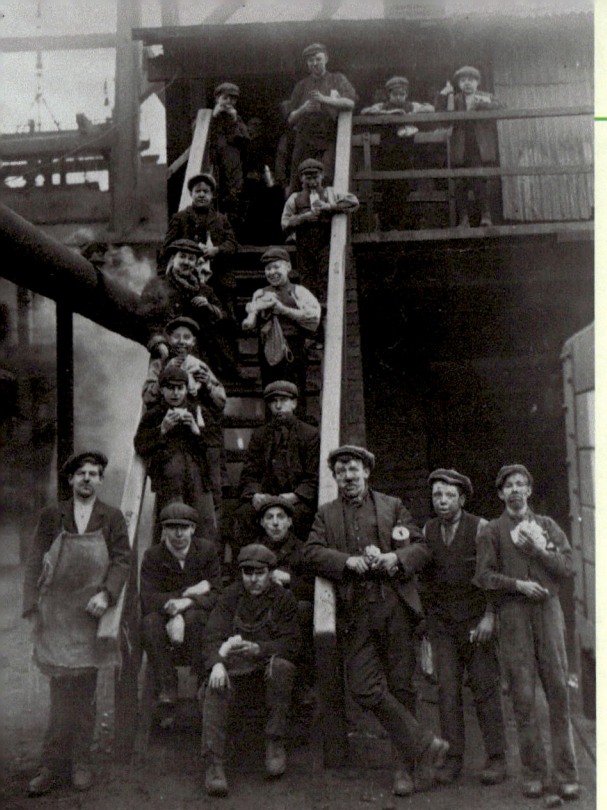

◀ Miners, young and old, at a Derbyshire coal mine in 1905

8. People and population c.1900

The population of Britain in 1900 was about 37 million. Well over half of these people lived in cities but farming was still a very important part of the country's wealth and way of life. Produce was still taken to market in towns and cities as it had been for centuries, although trains allowed fresh foodstuffs and other agricultural goods to be transported further, at speed. Richer families owned the land and relied on agricultural labourers to work in the fields, although the very first British tractors went on sale in 1901. These were to change country life forever as fewer labourers were needed and more families moved from villages to cities to find work throughout the century.

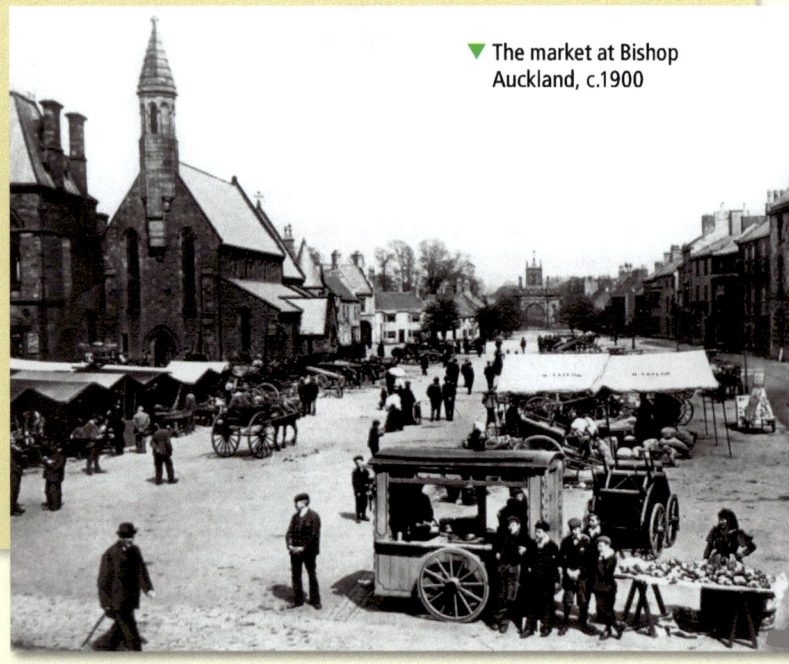

▼ The market at Bishop Auckland, c.1900

9. Leisure and lifestyle c.1900

Although the average worker did 54 hours per week, this still left Saturday afternoons and Sundays free. Leisure hours might be spent outside playing games such as football, walking in newly made public parks or working on an allotment. Others preferred to spend their time in a pub. Even if people did choose to sit drinking in pubs in their times of leisure, their general way of life often involved a lot of exercise as they walked from place to place and did most tasks, at work and at home, through their own muscle power.

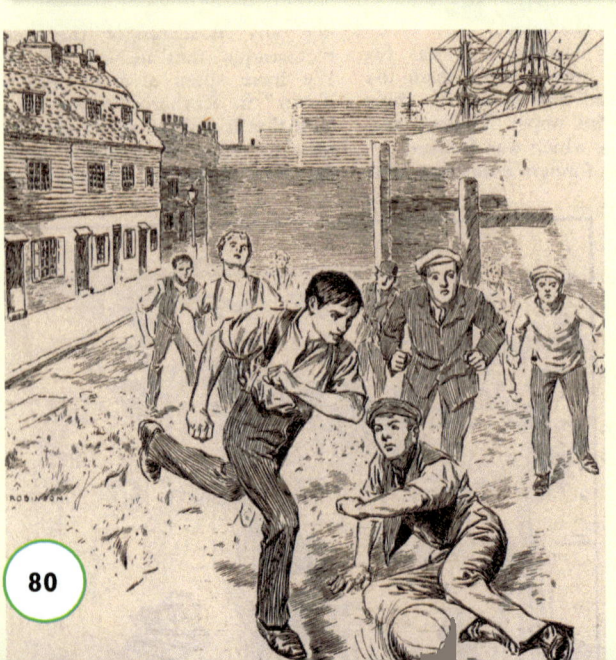

◀ Young men playing football in the street. From a magazine, c.1904

Do the changes in public health since 1900 tell a simple story of progress?

10. Work and wealth c.2000

Ever since the first steps towards a Welfare State in 1906, governments have raised taxes to pay for the pensions and other benefits that the state now provides. These taxes, as well as improvements in education, have changed the distribution of wealth in British society. By 2000, Britain had a much larger middle class. Most people have far more comfortable lives now than their great grandparents had in 1900. The British economy changed greatly, especially after about 1950. Jobs in mines, shipyards and factories disappeared thanks to changes in technology and competition from other nations. New jobs appeared in what are called 'service industries'. These include tourism, education, health care and finance. New technology in the home and improved methods of family planning freed women to take many of these jobs.

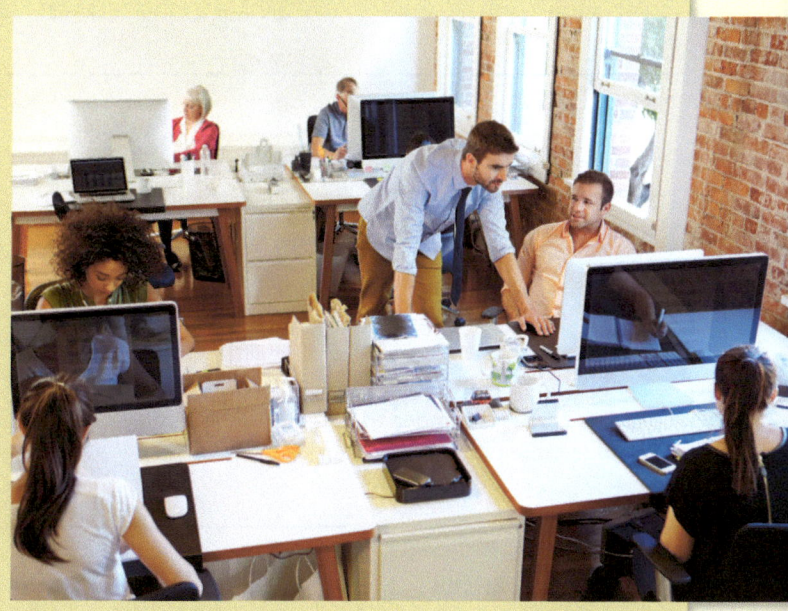

▶ Office work at the start of the twenty-first century

11. People and population c.2000

The population of Britain in 2000 was about 58 million and more people than ever now live in cities. Cities now have a far wider mix of ethnic groups as many Commonwealth citizens moved to Britain in the second half of the century to find work. These groups often moved into the poorer areas of cities when they first arrived and faced difficult living conditions. The growth in Britain's population led to a growth in the number of jobs and in the nation's wealth. It also put extra demands on the Welfare State, especially as separations and divorces became more common and more households were made up of single-parent families.

◀ A busy shopping centre in London, c.2012

12. Leisure and lifestyle c.2000

By 2000, the average working week was 39 hours and people were getting far more generous holidays. Together with the increased wealth enjoyed by most in society and great changes in technology, this has led to a huge growth in the leisure industry. People now spend time and money travelling, enjoying music, films and sport in ways that their ancestors could never have dreamed of. For many this involves participation and activity but others settle for being spectators in their own homes through televisions and other electronic devices.

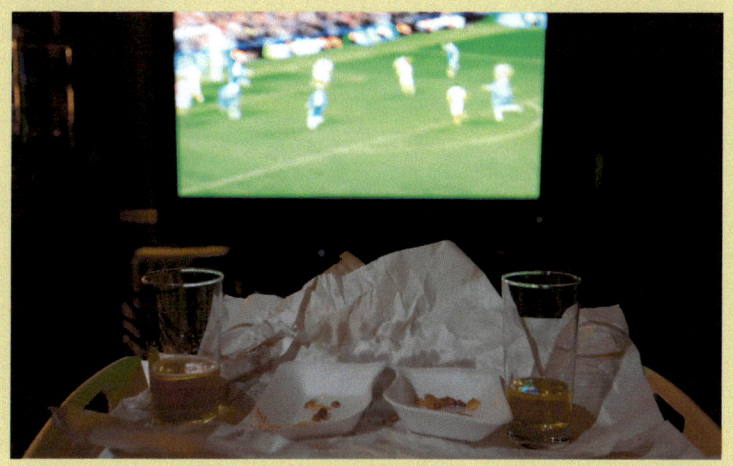

▶ A typical television fast-food dinner

Living conditions

Record

On the next six pages you will learn about four different aspects of living conditions in Britain between 1900 and the present day. They are:

- Housing
- Food
- Air
- Inactivity

As you read, remember to add new ideas and evidence to your table. Start with 'Housing'.

Issue	On the one hand there were signs of progress such as ...	On the other hand there were still significant challenges such as ...
Housing		

A letter from Bristol Council to a woman who was about to move from slum housing to a newly built council house in 1936

The Housing Committee realise that in worn out houses it is very difficult to get rid of vermin. But there will be no excuse in your new house. Do not buy second hand furniture, bedding or pictures unless you are quite sure that the articles are free from vermin. Insects do not like soap and hot water, and they also dislike dusters and polish. So if in your new house you keep your windows open, and keep your bodies and clothing, floors and stairs, furniture and bedding clean you are not likely to be troubled again with vermin.

Reflect

Why might the woman who received this letter have resented the advice it gives?

Housing

As you saw on page 77, many of Britain's poorest families were still living in unhealthy houses in 1900. The worst conditions were found in the terraced streets of back-to-back houses owned by private landlords who rented them out to working-class families.

In the first half of the twentieth century, governments took more and more responsibility for the people's health and this led them to tackle the nation's housing problems. The first step came in 1909 when Parliament banned any new back-to-back building. Private landowners and builders grumbled at this interference but it led to an improvement in privately owned housing.

The really big change came with Parliament's Housing Act of 1919. This

- ordered councils to become landlords for people living in poverty by building new, rented housing for working-class people in their area
- used taxpayers' money to help fund each local authority's building programme
- set standards for space, water supply and drainage that all new houses had to meet. Since then these have developed over time to control the quality of building materials as well as damp-proofing, ventilation, ceiling heights and window sizes.

These council houses were sometimes called 'homes fit for heroes' as the Prime Minister, Lloyd George, promised to build a 'country fit for heroes to live in' when troops returned to Britain after the war.

In 1921, work started on the Becontree Estate in Dagenham. By 1932, it had over 25,000 new houses which became homes for people from the east end of London. The council selected the new tenants from what it believed to be the 'more responsible' members of the working classes. The houses had inside toilets and bathrooms. As they were now landlords, each local authority set up a housing committee to oversee its new council houses and to ensure they were well maintained.

Despite such developments, the worst slums remained, often with the poorest families of all still living in them. Governments could see that private landlords were not going to build new houses for the poorest families. So, in 1930, it passed another Housing Act. This took a brave new approach: it allowed councils to force private landlords to sell their houses in the slums to the council. The councils could then clear the slums and use the land to build new, clean homes.

Do the changes in public health since 1900 tell a simple story of progress?

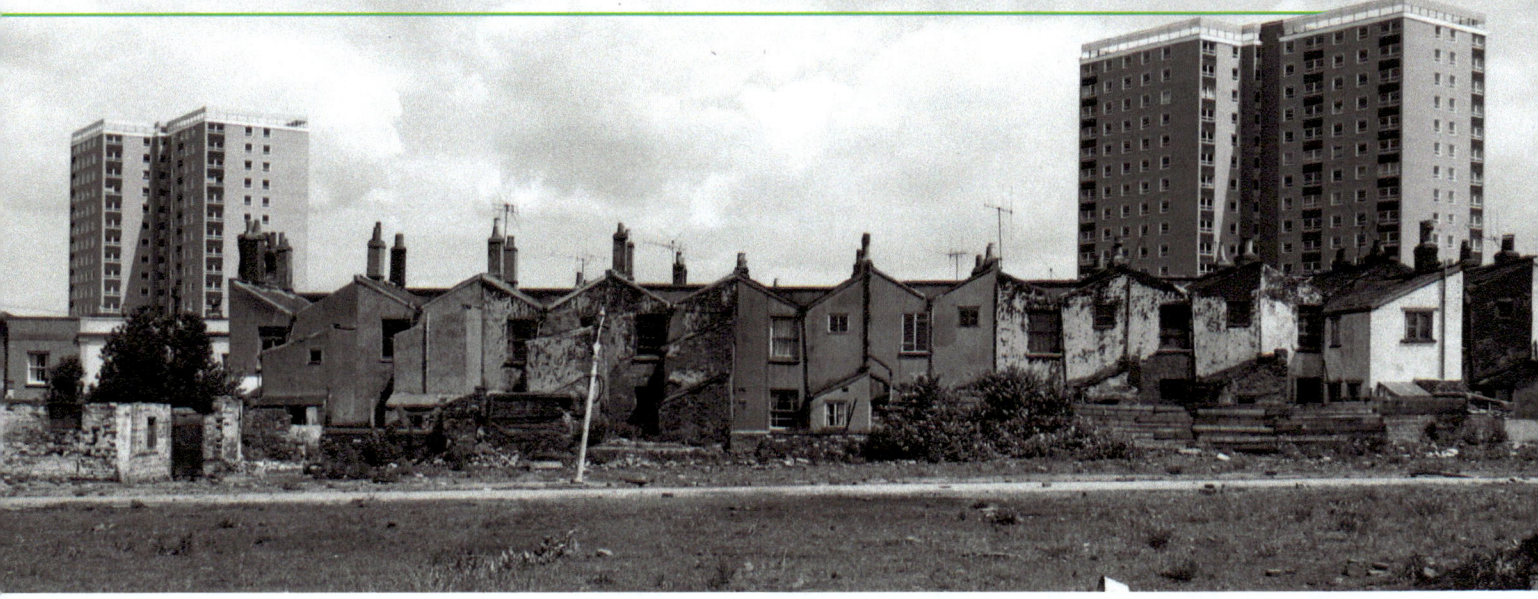

▲ Bristol in the 1960s – high-rise council flats overlooking the back-to-back housing they replaced

Streets in the air

City councils wanted to build as many homes as they could on the land they bought. The development of gas and electric heaters and cookers meant that householders no longer needed to store or move coal. This allowed local authorities to start building low-rise blocks of flats, three or four storeys high.

By the end of the Second World War in 1945, bomb damage had destroyed about 475,000 houses in Britain's cities. The next three decades saw an enormous programme of council-house building. At first, most were houses, but in the 1960s and 1970s governments offered more generous funding to councils who built flats over six-storeys high. Developments in automated lifts meant that flats could go 'high-rise' and building upwards meant that councils did not need to find new land beyond the city. 4,500 tower blocks had been built by 1980. Many of the people who moved from back-to-back housing into high-rise flats appreciated the modern facilities but became lonely and depressed away from the neighbourhood communities they had grown up in.

Decline of council housing

By 1979, 42 per cent of the population lived in council housing of some sort compared with just 1 per cent in 1900. The Conservative Prime Minister, Margaret Thatcher, thought things had gone too far. She believed people would be less dependent on the state if they owned their own homes. In 1980, she passed a Housing Act that gave tenants the right to buy their council homes. Since then about 1.5 million council homes have been sold to tenants, especially those in houses. This left councils with fewer houses for families in need of shelter. Government restrictions on council spending meant that they could not replace the houses that were sold. This has led to a rise in renting from private landlords. This can work very well, but reports in the last decade have revealed that over 50 per cent of private rented housing failed to meet the government's required standards for healthy homes as set out in 2000. They had problems with one or more of damp, mould, excessive cold, poor lighting or other issues that may cause accidents.

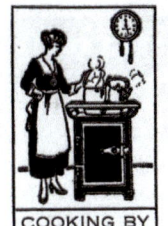

▲ An advert for electric cookers from the 1920s

> **The World Health Organisation's definition of health, issued in 1948. Britain has signed up to use this definition in its own health policies**
>
> Health is a state of complete physical, mental and social well-being and not merely the absence of disease or infirmity.

Reflect

Do you think government policies on housing since 1945 help Britain to be healthy according to this definition by the World Health Organisation?

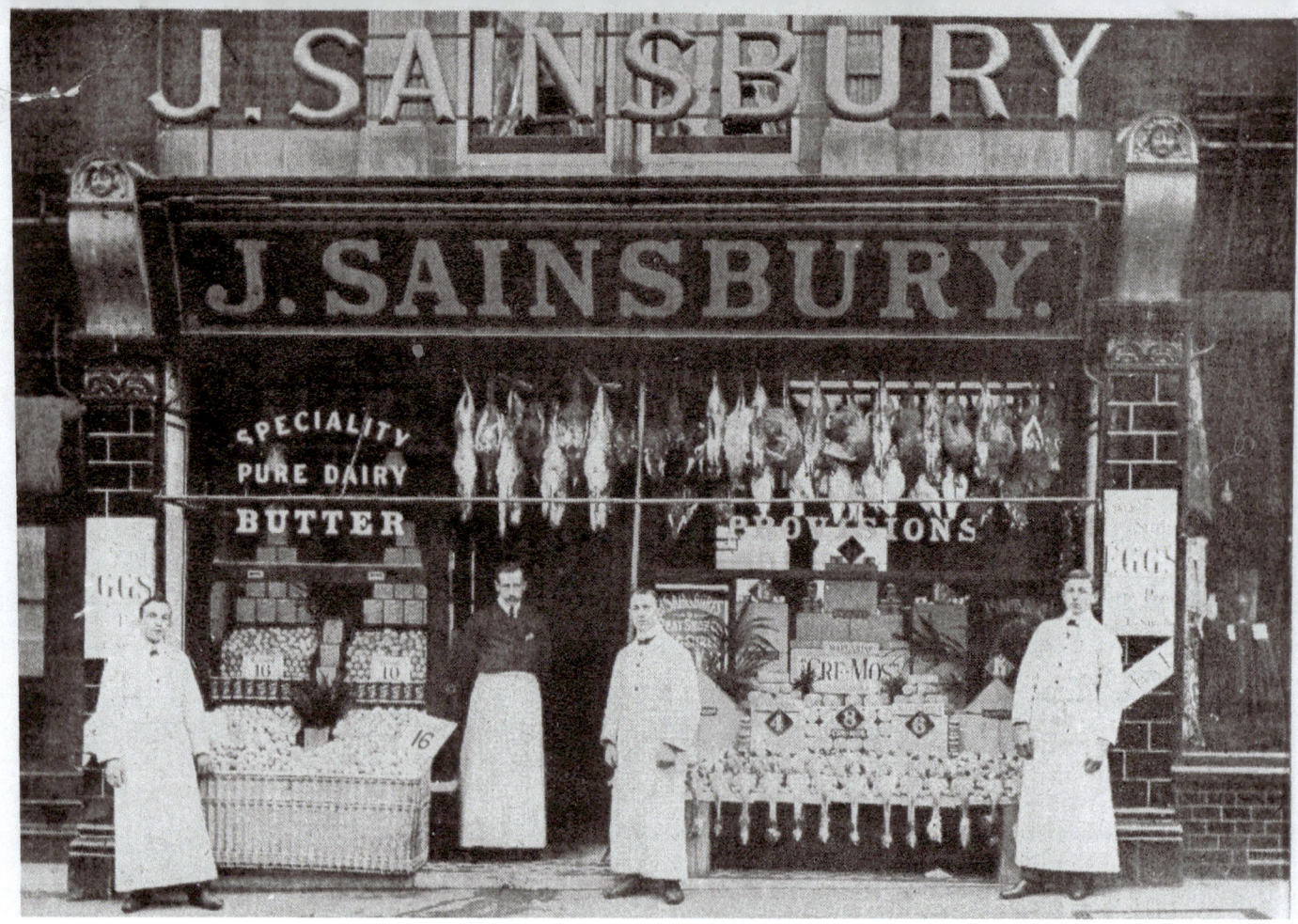

▲ A Sainsbury's shop in 1904

Food

The last twenty-five years of the nineteenth century saw important changes in Britain's food supply. From 1875, the government began to take a grip on food adulteration. Scientific advances made it easier to identify additives such as chalk and the fact that working men could vote probably made the politicians more ready to take action to make sure the food these men were eating was of reasonable quality.

At the same time, science and technology also improved food supply. Ships carried cheap wheat from North America and refrigerated lamb from New Zealand. New methods of grinding grain produced bread that was purer and easier to eat. The canning of foods became more reliable and the first tin of Heinz baked beans went on sale in 1905. Condensed milk kept for up to a year unlike natural milk. Margarine was a cheap substitute for butter.

The way food was sold and bought also changed around 1900. Chains of grocery stores such as Sainsbury's and Lipton's became popular. Unlike the old style markets, they were open every day and had regular and reliable stocks. For most people these were really helpful changes, especially as the wages of skilled workers were rising just as the price of these foodstuffs was falling. Items that would have been luxuries long ago became more common. Chocolates, sweets, biscuits and jams were easily affordable for many. In 1914, a working family in Britain spent about 60 per cent of its income on food. By 1937, this had fallen to 37 per cent.

> ### Reflect
> How is this Sainsbury's shop trying to mix the feel of an old-fashioned market with modern, efficient shop-keeping?

The impact of war

The outbreak of the Second World War in 1939 upset this pattern. It became almost impossible to import goods from abroad and every effort went into producing as much food as possible on British farms. The government introduced food rationing and tried to ensure that whatever food was available was nourishing and fairly distributed. People missed their sweets and foreign fruit but those with a patch of land could grow their own vegetables or keep animals such as pigs, chickens and rabbits as their ancestors had done for centuries. The war ended in 1945 but rationing continued until 1954. The health of Britain's poor actually improved under rationing as they were eating a more balanced diet.

Do the changes in public health since 1900 tell a simple story of progress?

The impact of wealth

Changes in Britain's food supply accelerated after 1950 as most families became richer. In 1959, thirteen per cent of homes had a refrigerator. Now almost every household has one as well as a freezer. More women went out to work and families increasingly relied on ready-made meals. Manufacturers added various preservatives to these meals to give them a longer shelf life. Some dishes reflected Britain's increasingly diverse population, as immigrants came seeking work after 1945, and changing tastes as more people travelled abroad and enjoyed foreign food. The microwave cooker was invented in the USA in the 1950s and, by 1975, it was outselling gas cookers in Britain. Convenience food was becoming part of the nation's lifestyle.

> ### Reflect
> Why do you think relatively few poor families buy so-called 'health foods' and fresh fruit and vegetables?

New fears about food

Britain has faced a series of health scares over its food since the 1980s. In 1986 a new disease known as BSE infected the brains of cows. The government's scientists insisted for years that this could not be transferred to humans who ate meat from the infected animals but in 1996 they admitted that they were mistaken. Sales of beef products plummeted until new systems identified and destroyed all animals with BSE.

In recent years some people have avoided buying processed foods and try to eat only the freshest produce available, even if it is more expensive. They are concerned that modern farming and food production is done on an industrial scale. They point out, for example, that the feed now given to most farm animals contains antibiotics. This is to keep the animals healthy and help them grow, but as humans eat the meat and drink the milk from these animals, traces of antibiotics pass into our bodies. This allows germs that could once be killed by antibiotics to develop a resistance. Our modern diet may be sending us back to the days before the first antibiotics, when a minor infection could kill us.

Children's food and health – a case study

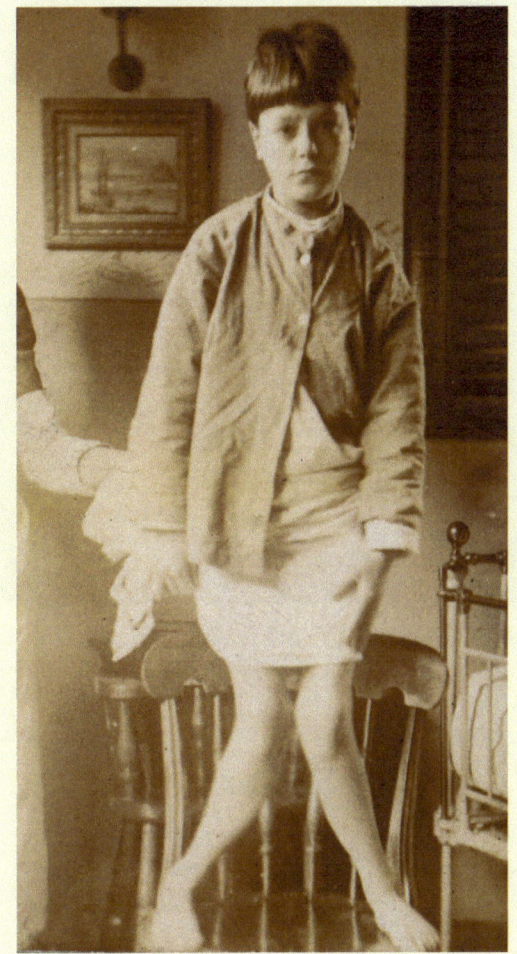

◀ A boy with rickets, c.1900

This young boy is just one of the many thousands of young people living in 1900 who suffered from a disease called rickets. When the body fails to get enough vitamin D, either from food or from exposure to sunlight, the bones become weak and twisted. People had suffered from rickets for centuries but in 1900 the problem was worse than ever in the poorer areas of Britain's towns.

Rickets affected so many in 1900 because people living in poverty were changing their diet. They ate far less fresh fruit and fish and some drank sweetened condensed milk. The new way of grinding grain removed many of its most valuable vitamins. It was only in 1942 that scientists recommended adding extra vitamins to bread to make up for this. The other problem was that the body needs sunlight to build up its vitamin D. In 1900, many children like this boy were living in dark houses, down dark alleys, in dark cities.

Given all the changes in housing and food, you might imagine that rickets is no longer a problem in Britain. However, in 2014 doctors reported an alarming rise in the disease in young people. Over reliance on processed foods and takeaway meals is leading, once again, to malnutrition and lack of vitamin D, especially among poorer communities. Children are also spending far less time outdoors as they play on computers and watch television so they are missing the exposure to sunlight that their bodies need, even though they almost certainly live in far healthier houses than this boy knew in 1900.

Air

Problems from coal

In 1800, Britain consumed around 10 million tons of coal each year. By 1950, that figure had risen to 200 million tons. The skies above cities such as Glasgow, Manchester, Leeds and London were almost permanently filled with a haze of smoke from factory and household chimneys. In 1853, 1875 and 1926, laws were passed that allowed the police to prosecute offending factory owners, but they were very rarely used. In some ways Britain saw the smoke-filled skies over its cities as a badge of honour, a sign of the nation's booming economy. People could not accept that coal fires should be banned just as most drivers today would resist any ban on the use of motor cars.

There were times, though, when the problem of pollution was impossible to ignore. In certain conditions, usually in the winter, this smoke became trapped under a thick blanket of fog that could last for days on end. In 1905, someone invented a new word for this problem – 'smog'. The air became so thick with sulphur that people with weak lungs and heart could not get enough oxygen into their bodies. They might develop pneumonia or bronchitis or they might collapse and die in the street after straining to breath.

Between 4 and 12 December 1952, London suffered the worst smog it had ever known. It is estimated that it killed about 12,000 Londoners. The government knew that it had to act and in 1956 it passed the Clean Air Act. This required factories and homes in specified areas to burn special types of 'smokeless' fuel. Slowly these smokeless zones grew, helped by the arrival of improved oil, gas and electric heating systems. By the 1980s, smog was no longer a problem. Or so it seemed …

Problems from cars

Smoke from coal fires may have been disappearing but exhaust fumes from motor vehicles have created a new version of the old problem. Car ownership in Britain increased by over a quarter between 1980 and 1990 and has continued to rise since. When scientists discovered that petrol engines used to release poisonous lead into the air, new laws were brought in to force oil companies to make lead-free fuel. From 2001, governments encouraged motorists to buy diesel engine vehicles, believing they would cause fewer problems as they use less fuel. Since then, scientists have shown that diesel engines may actually cause more harm as they emit tiny particles into the air that may, in certain circumstances, cause cancer. Whether from petrol or diesel engines, London and other large cities are now experiencing smog once again. This time the cause is not coal, but exhaust fumes. In 2014 and again in 2015, athletes in London were warned not to go out training in the weeks before the London marathon as there were dangerously high levels of pollutants in the air over London.

> **Reflect**
> How does smoke pollution help to explain why so many children suffered from rickets by 1900?

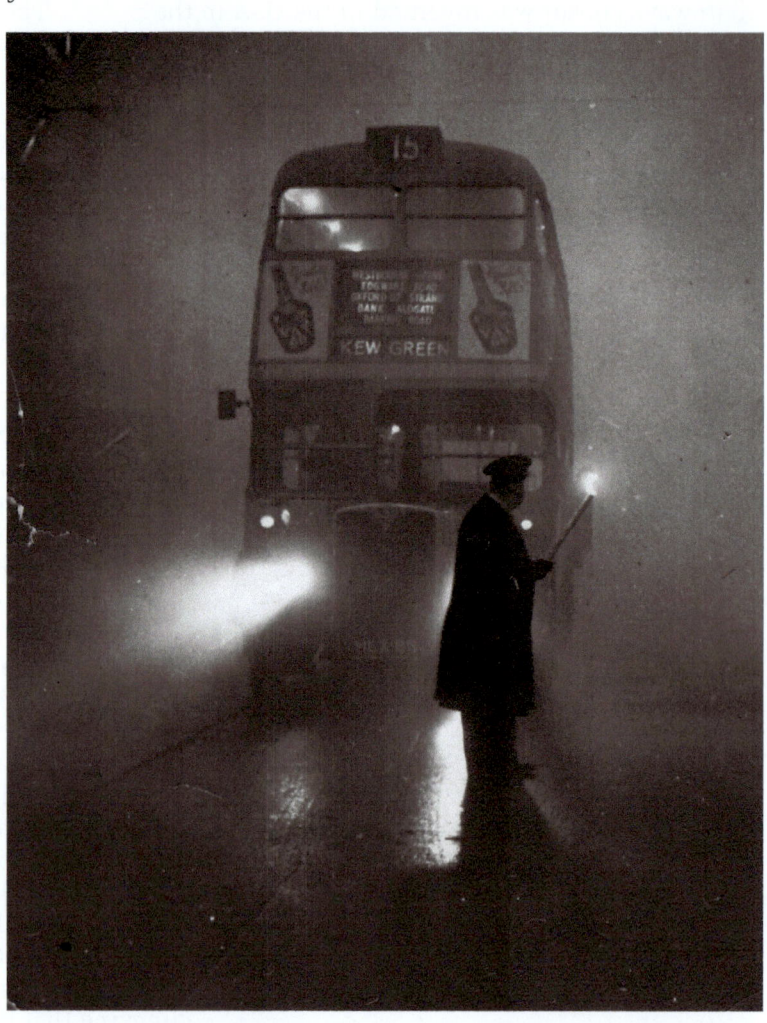

▲ A policeman guides a bus along a London street at walking pace during the great smog of 1952

> **Reflect**
> What do you think would happen if science ever proved that diesel exhaust fumes do cause cancer?

Inactivity

Problems from consuming

The artist who drew this cartoon in 2008 seems to be clear that a lot has changed over the last century! The three figures on the left trace human evolution over millions of years. The two figures on the right show the artist's view of how people have changed in just the last hundred years or so, since the time of the First World War.

In 1914, when that war started, the nation was, in general terms, wealthy. Levels of exercise dropped as growing numbers of people paid to use trains and trams. The millions who had regular work spent their rising wages on non-essentials including sweeter foods. The Industrial Revolution had already created all sorts of labour-saving devices for factories and homes. Traders were becoming expert at selling these and other goods through carefully crafted advertisements. These were the ingredients that have led to the change shown in the cartoon. People were becoming 'consumers'.

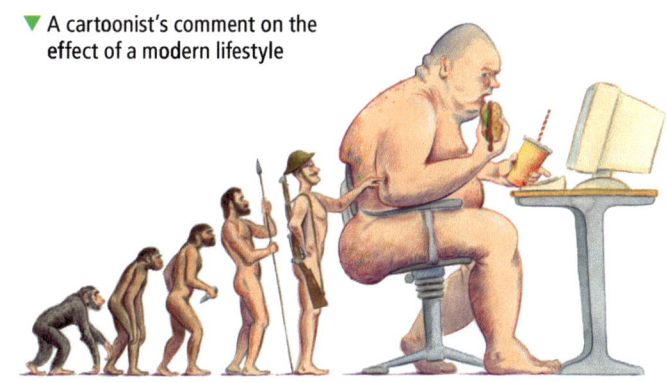

A cartoonist's comment on the effect of a modern lifestyle

More problems from cars

By the 1920s, the government's chief medical officer was concerned that many Britons were becoming unhealthy through 'excessive and unsuitable food, combined with lack of fresh air and exercise'. By this time, motor cars had taken over from horse-drawn transport, and this may already have been affecting the exercise levels of those who owned them. In the late 1920s and 1930s, middle-class magazines were full of articles and advertisements about slimming. These disappeared during the Second World War when working hours were longer, and both food and petrol were rationed. People were far more active, walking everywhere and digging their gardens to grow vegetables.

Of course, governments knew they could not control people's behaviour in the same way when peace returned in 1945. After the end of rationing in 1954, the middle-class lifestyle that worried the chief medical officer in the 1920s spread throughout all groups in society.

New technology has accelerated the changes in the way we live:

- We watch television or use tablets as we sit on our sofas.
- We use remote controls to switch TV channels without moving from our seats.
- Far more people watch sport on television than take part in it.
- Power tools and household appliances mean jobs in our homes that once involved effort are now far less physically demanding.
- Robots do the heavy work in factories while workers watch monitors.

A research project in 2013 showed that the poorer parts of society are the least active. Almost three-quarters of people who have no qualifications take little or no exercise. Overall, 44 per cent of men and 33 per cent of women were classified as overweight. This is a strange contrast with the position just before the First World War. In the 1890s, 40 per cent of men from industrial towns were found to be too weak to be allowed to join the army; in 2006 over a third of the nation's teenagers would have been too fat to be allowed to join up, so the army changed its standards and accepted volunteers who, until then, would have been classed as overweight.

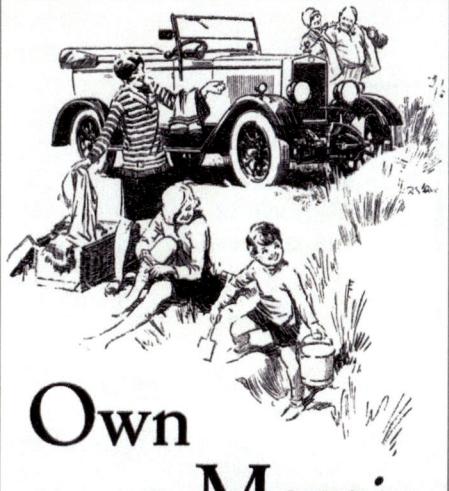

▲ An advertisement for a Morris car in the 1920s

Record

Remember to add ideas and evidence to your table (see page 82).

Responses to epidemics

> ### Record
> Louis Pasteur's discovery that germs cause infectious diseases led to the development of vaccines that now immunise people against many of the nineteenth-century's killer diseases. But the twentieth century saw outbreaks of two new and deadly epidemics. As you read about each one, add more notes to your table. (See page 82.)

The Spanish flu

Between 1914 and 1918, approximately 17 million people across the world died as casualties of the First World War. Between 1918 and 1919, at least 50 million died as a result of a less well-known global disaster, the Spanish influenza epidemic. In Britain alone it killed 228,000. It took more lives in one year than the Black Death had done between 1348 and 1351.

The disease is called Spanish influenza (or Spanish flu) simply because the first widely reported cases in Europe were in Spain, but it struck almost every nation on Earth. By early 1918, it was rife in the trenches of northern Europe. Soldiers then spread the infection to Britain when they returned on leave. The first wave in Britain lasted from June to July 1918. It then died down before surging back for its most devastating attack from October to December. It reached its peak just at the end of the war on 11 November as people celebrated in enormous crowds. It faded again but returned between February and May 1919.

> ### Reflect
> How did the ending of the First World War help to spread Spanish flu?

The symptoms of Spanish flu caused great alarm. It would start with signs of a common cold or flu such as a chill, high temperature, headache and pains in the back and limbs. For some, the symptoms stopped there and they survived. For others, it turned into a vicious attack of pneumonia. Blue patches and dark spots appeared on their cheeks, indicating that the body was struggling to get enough oxygen. They might have bled from the nose, ears or stomach as they fought to take in air. Someone could be healthy in the morning and dead by teatime.

No one knew what caused the Spanish flu. Practical experience and new discoveries about germs meant that people used face masks to avoid breathing air that might have been infected by the breath of flu victims.

We now know that Spanish flu started as a virus that affects birds. This jumped to infect humans, probably in the Far East. It was then carried to Europe by labourers brought from China to work in army camps in France during the war. From there, the disease ran riot.

We still do not know how to cure influenza today although there are vaccines that offer some protection. A new flu virus could attack the world at any time. For all our scientific advances, we would still be largely defenceless.

▼ A woman wearing an expensive home air-filter in 1919

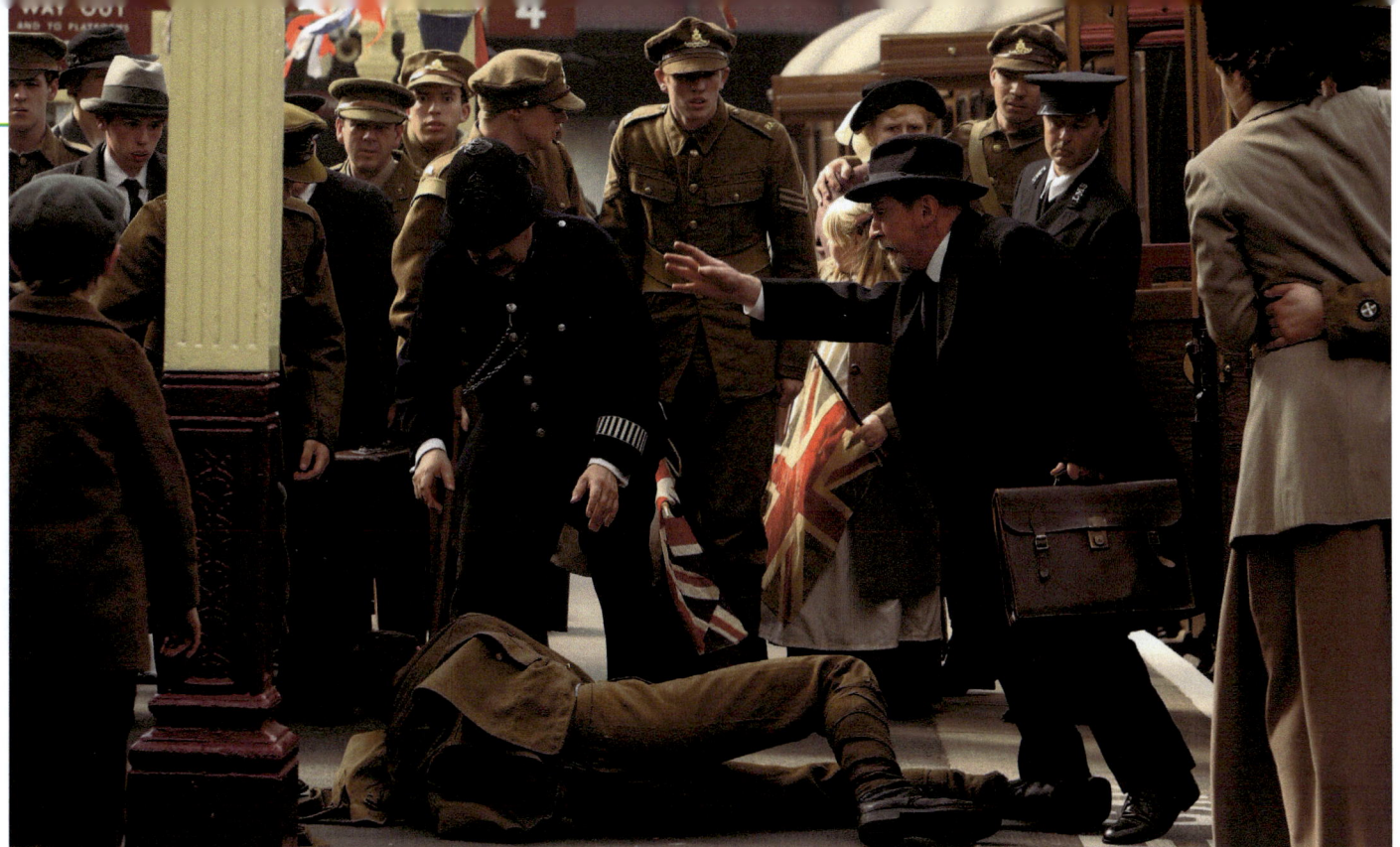

▲ In this still from the BBC drama 'The Forgotten Fallen', Doctor Niven is urging everyone to step back from a soldier who has just returned from France and has collapsed on the platform.

Doctor Niven of Manchester and the Spanish flu

As you learned on page 71, the 1875 Public Health Act required each town to appoint a medical officer. In 1918, Manchester's medical officer was Dr James Niven. The BBC made a television drama about him in 2009. It shows how he worked tirelessly to limit the impact of the epidemic on the city.

In 1919, Dr Niven wrote a very thorough report on the Spanish influenza. The list below shows some of the actions he took while the epidemic was raging in Manchester and how others around him responded.

- He kept detailed records of each flu victim's case and looked for patterns about who was affected, when and where.
- He praised the efforts of the nurses and doctors who risked their lives by treating the sick.
- He sent health visitors door to door to record on special cards who was ill and what help they needed, for example, coal or food.
- He referred to records of earlier severe flu outbreaks.
- He arranged for extra grave-diggers to be appointed.
- He published detailed advice in newspapers.
- He recommended to the government that they must invest money into researching colds and influenza.
- He visited factories and schools to see for himself how the disease first affected its victims and to advise on how to avoid it.
- He used his medical contacts to try a new flu vaccine. It did not work.
- He urged the council to shut all schools but it was slow to follow his advice.
- He insisted that theatres and cinemas could only stay open if they had good ventilation and were disinfected between shows.
- He issued flu advice leaflets, insisting on regular hand-washing, using handkerchiefs and wearing face masks, for example, when on buses.
- He arranged for a film about the flu to be shown in cinemas.
- He used simple language to give the public advice, for example, 'spit kills'.

Dr Niven's determination to limit the spread of Spanish influenza in Manchester seems to have worked. Two thousand people died there but the proportion was much higher in cities such as Glasgow and London. In his report, Dr Niven said that, in future, people might expect greater protection from public health officials like him. He suffered from depression after he retired and in 1926 he committed suicide.

Reflect
1. Which of Dr Niven's actions would you put under each of these headings:
   - research
   - practical action
   - publicity?
2. Which three of his actions do you think did most to help the people of Manchester?

AIDS

In the 1970s, doctors in Europe, North America and Africa encountered a strange new medical condition. Victims suffered from pneumonia, severe weight loss and sores on their skin. Their bodies wasted and they died. No one could explain this and it went unreported in the media. Then, in 1981, five gay men in Los Angeles and one in Britain died from the condition. It appeared to be caused by a problem with the body's immune system. In 1982, it was given the name AIDS – Acquired Immune Deficiency Syndrome.

AIDS itself is not a disease, it is just a condition where the victim's natural defences can no longer fight off other infections. In 1984, scientists discovered the virus that causes AIDS. In 1986, they named it HIV – Human Immunodeficiency Virus. Unlike other epidemics we have studied, this virus cannot be spread through the air or simply by touch. Over time, doctors discovered that it is spread through blood or body fluids, for example by:

- sexual contact with an infected person
- sharing **hypodermic** needles with an infected person
- receiving a blood transfusion using blood from an infected person
- being a child in the womb of an infected mother.

Society's response to HIV/AIDS can be divided into five main phases.

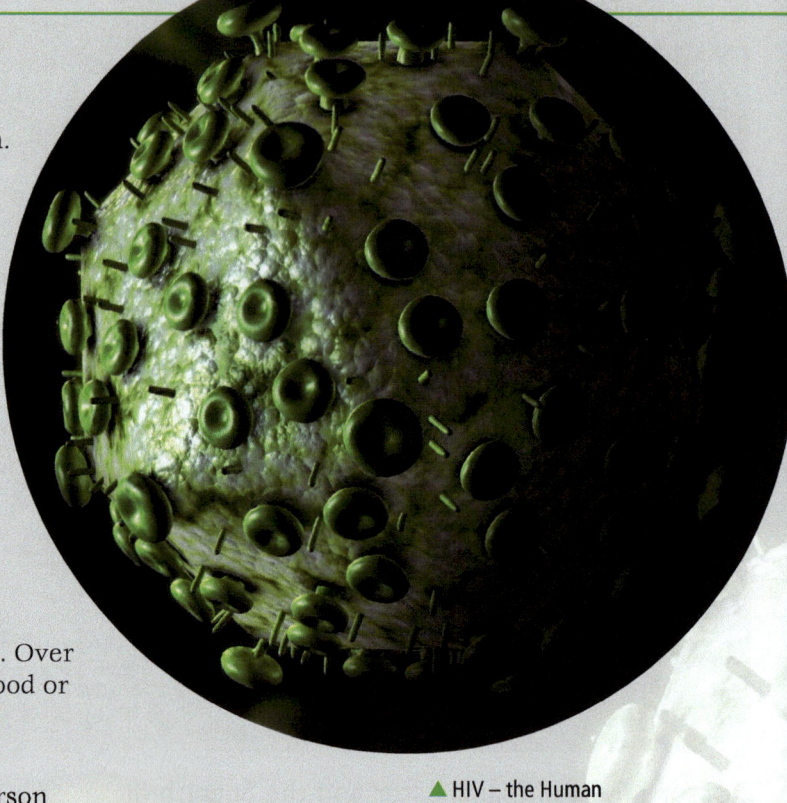

▲ HIV – the Human Immunodeficiency Virus, greatly magnified

Phase 1 (1970s–1983) – Growing awareness

By 1982, seven people in Britain had died from AIDS. Friends of one of these set up the Terrence Higgins Trust to raise funds for research and to raise awareness of the illness, but very few people shared their concern over AIDS at this stage.

The media first took an interest in 1983 when a number of people developed AIDS after receiving a blood transfusion. The government urged groups it identified as being particularly at risk from AIDS, including gay people and drug addicts, to stop donating blood. One newspaper ran a story about 'Killer Blood' in British hospitals and soon afterwards two television documentaries about AIDS were made. They emphasised that the condition was normally associated with gay men. One newspaper article used the headline 'Gay Plague'.

Early reporting of AIDS often led to discrimination. Many people argued that AIDS was not like cholera or the Spanish flu as it could and should be avoided if men would refrain from having sex with other men and if drug users would kick their habit. Some Church leaders preached that AIDS was God's punishment on gay people and drug addicts.

Phase 2 (1984–85) – Growing alarm

People were unsure how easily AIDS could spread and over reacted:

- Some Fire Service staff stopped giving mouth-to-mouth resuscitation for fear of infection.
- Some churchgoers refused to share the cup from which everyone drank wine at the service of Holy Communion.
- Parents withdrew their children from a class when one pupil acquired HIV through a blood transfusion.

There was no risk of getting AIDS from any of these situations, but at the time this was not made clear.

> **Reflect**
>
> Why were so many people deeply alarmed about AIDS in these first two phases?

People's fears increased in 1985 when the Royal College of Nursing wrongly predicted that Britain would have one million cases of AIDS by 1991. The government caused alarm by ordering hospitals to detain patients with AIDS even if they wished to leave. Doctors and visitors had to wear gowns, masks and gloves, which reinforced fears that AIDS could be spread by the slightest contact.

Phase 3 (1986–87) – Growing understanding

By this time, more helpful actions were under way:

- Charity groups, including some run by churches, provided clean needles to drug addicts to reduce cross-infection.
- The government funded free testing for HIV at hospitals and the screening of all blood donations so blood transfusions were safe.
- The government also organised an AIDS prevention campaign. It sent a leaflet called 'Don't die of ignorance' to every home in Britain and ran advertisements on television on how to avoid contracting AIDS.
- Television programmes, poster campaigns and radio phone-in shows helped to end myths about how AIDS spread.
- The real breakthrough came in April 1987 when Princess Diana, the most famous and popular member of the Royal family at the time, visited a clinic and made sure that news reports showed photographs of her shaking hands with someone who was suffering from AIDS. People were reassured that AIDS could not be passed on by simple contact and that those who suffered from it deserved compassion and respect.

Phase 4 (1988–95) – Growing acceptance

The late 1980s and early 1990s were years when AIDS became more widely understood. In 1991, a storyline was included in the BBC television series *Eastenders* about a character who was diagnosed HIV-positive. In the same year the enormously popular rock star, Freddie Mercury, died from AIDS. In 1992, a tribute concert and a special release of one of his greatest hits raised around £20 million for AIDS causes. This would have been unthinkable a few years beforehand. AIDS was spreading, but at nothing like the rate that had been predicted by the Royal College of Nursing. Measures to make blood transfusions safe and advice about safe sex and not sharing needles was working. By 1995, about 25,000 people in Britain had been diagnosed HIV-positive. Twelve thousand of these had developed AIDS and around 8,500 of these people had died.

Phase 5 (from 1996) – Growing complacency

In 1996 came unexpected news: scientists had devised drugs called 'anti-retrovirals' that delayed the onset of AIDS in people infected with HIV. These were very expensive but the government funded them. This was very good news but it has had unexpected consequences.

The government relaxed its campaigns about AIDS and HIV. Many people believe these anti-retrovirals are a 'cure' for AIDS and this has led to complacency. Instead of falling, cases of HIV infection, as well as a range of other sexually transmitted diseases, have risen alarmingly in recent years. In 2009 there were about 100,000 people in Britain living with HIV. Of these, 40,000, were gay men and the rest were heterosexual men and women. About a quarter of all those with HIV are not aware of their condition and may be spreading the infection without knowing it.

Far from helping to end this epidemic, the discovery of an effective treatment seems to have made it worse.

Reflect

Which of the actions listed here do you think was most likely to help people understand AIDS better?

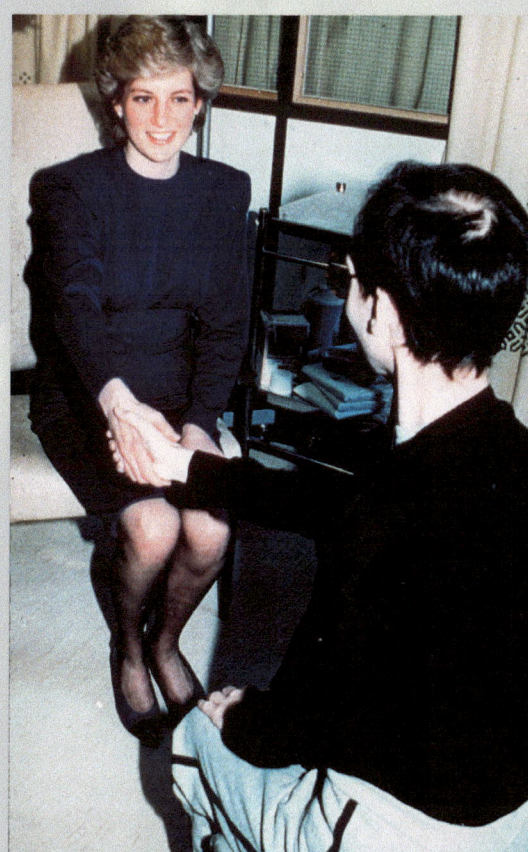

▼ Princess Diana's famous handshake with an AIDS patient in April 1987

Record

Remember to add ideas and evidence to your table. (See page 82.)

Growing government involvement

Laws

As you will already have seen in this enquiry, the government has become more and more closely involved with looking after the people's health since 1900. This diagram shows just a few of the main landmarks in government legislation across the twentieth century. Read the information by working clockwise from 1902.

▼ Landmarks in public health legislation since 1900

> **Record**
> Keep looking for signs of progress and signs of remaining challenges. Add them to your table. (See page 82.)

1902 Regulation and training of midwives

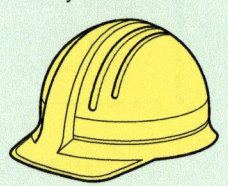

1906 Free school meals for very poor children

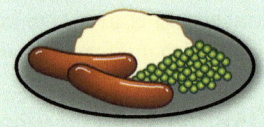

1907 Medical inspections at school

1908 Old age pensions for the over 70s

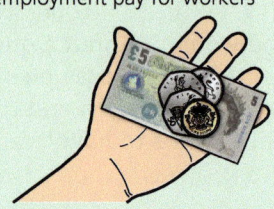

1911 National Insurance scheme to provide sickness and unemployment pay for workers

1919 Local authorities required to start slum clearance and council house building

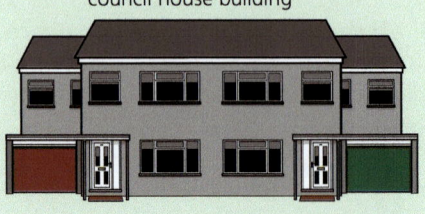

1929 Local authorities took over some old workhouse hospitals when the Poor Laws ended

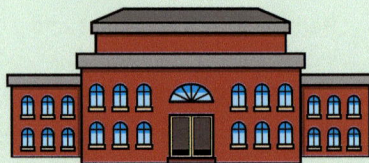

1940 Start of major immunisation programme:
- Diphtheria (1940)
- Tuberculosis (1948)

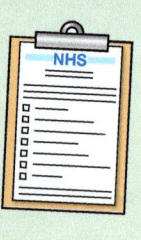

1948 National Health Service: hospital care, family doctors, dentists and medicines provided free. (Some charges have since been imposed.)

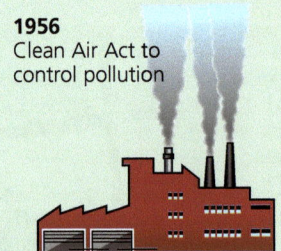

1956 Clean Air Act to control pollution

1974 Health and Safety at Work Act

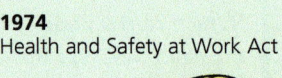

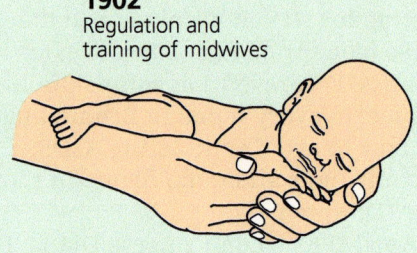

Houses of Parliament

Council offices

Do the changes in public health since 1900 tell a simple story of progress?

Sickness and health

In 1945, at the end of the Second World War, there was a general election in Britain. The Labour Party won by promising to defeat Britain's long-standing social problems in the same way the country had just defeated Nazi Germany. One of those long-standing problems was disease. This is why the new Labour government set up the National Health Service (NHS) in 1948.

The NHS is funded from taxpayers' money so that everyone in the country can receive treatment. Those with some personal wealth may pay extra charges, but the poorest are treated for free.

The services of the NHS have grown ever since it was created and, despite constant pressures on its staff and its systems, it provides an extraordinary range of care. It is, however, more concerned with treating those who are ill than with preventing disease. Some call it a 'National Sickness Service'.

Even though it is not given a high priority within the NHS, the work of the government in promoting public health has grown since 1945. It now spreads important information and advice to the public on an ever-increasing range of issues. Occasionally this has also led to direct government legislation as well. The best example concerns smoking.

Smoking

A harmless pleasure?

This advertisement appeared in 1952. It links smoking with the glamour of professional football. This would be unthinkable now, but in the 1950s the health hazards of tobacco were only just being discovered and smoking was part of everyday life. In the 1880s, machines were invented that rolled cigarettes automatically and made them much cheaper and more widely available. After 1947, the British government even offered free smoking tokens to pensioners to help them to buy cigarettes. By 1950, about 80 per cent of men and 40 per cent of women smoked.

But by this time, scientists already suspected that smoking caused cancer. They urged the government to protect people from the harmful effects of tobacco. Government ministers decided to take no action. The notes of their discussions included this statement:

> From the point of view of social health, cancer of the lung is not a disease like tuberculosis; nor should the government assume too lightly the position of advising the general public on their personal tastes and habits where the evidence of the harm is not conclusive.

The government clearly did not want to get involved before there was firm proof that smoking caused lung cancer. They lived in fear of taking the Welfare State too far and creating what has often been called a 'Nanny State', where a government takes responsibility away from individuals. This has been a concern ever since.

> **Reflect**
>
> Why do you think some people call the National Health Service a 'National Sickness Service'?

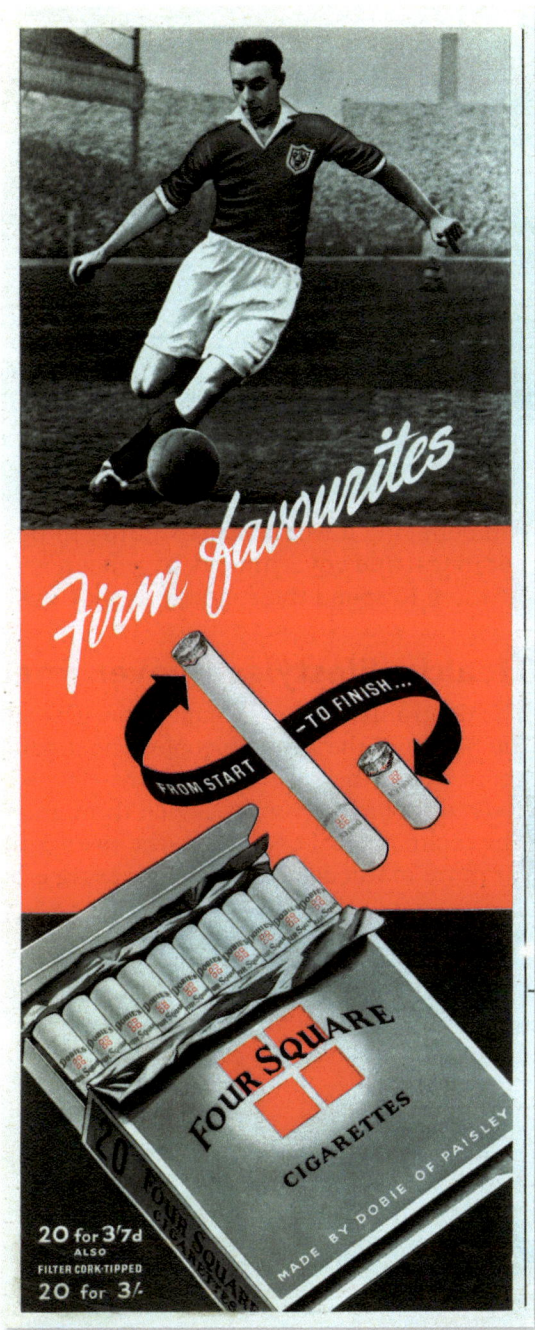

▲ A 1952 advert for cigarettes

> **Reflect**
>
> What does the term 'Nanny State' mean?

Time for action against smoking ... but slowly

In 1962, the Royal College of Physicians in London published 'Smoking and health', a document that provided convincing proof that smoking tobacco causes lung cancer and bronchitis. From that point onwards, steps have been taken to tackle these dangers.

- **1964** – Cigarette advertising was banned on television.
- **1971** – Government health warnings were printed on cigarette packs.
- **1986** – Cinema advertising of cigarettes was banned.
- **1998** – Government agreed to fund free nicotine replacement therapies for anyone trying to quit smoking.
- **2007** – Smoking was banned in all public places after a 2005 medical report showed that 'passive smoking' probably kills more than 11,000 people a year in Britain.
- **2016** – All cigarette packages to be blank with no attractive colours.

There were many reasons for the slow move towards ending tobacco smoking in Britain. Some say that governments know they need the income that is raised from the tax paid on every pack of cigarettes that is sold. The tobacco companies have naturally used their considerable wealth to defend their industry against restrictions. Some feared that a ban on smoking at work and other public places would increase smoking in the home which would threaten the health of children. Pubs and restaurants resisted this ban believing it would lead to a drop in their business. Above all, smoking is not illegal and governments have been very reluctant to restrict people's freedom to spend their money as they wish.

Reflect
Do you think the government should simply ban smoking completely?

Healthy lifestyles – government advice

The diagram on page 92 shows how government has passed laws to protect the health of the British people. The diagram below shows a range of issues about which the government gives advice. At the start of the century, it could only have given its advice through newspapers, posters and leaflets. The technological changes in the twentieth century mean that it now has far more methods of getting its messages across.

▼ Issues on which the government regularly provides advice to the public

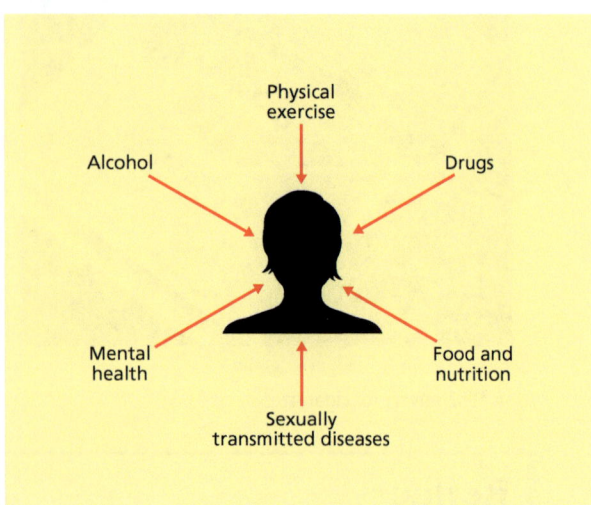

Reflect
1. Arrange the issues in the diagram in the order of importance that you think they should be given.
2. What different forms of communication does the government use today to spread its advice on health issues?

Do the changes in public health since 1900 tell a simple story of progress?

The cost of a healthy society

We started this enquiry by looking at the faces of some of London's poor and thinking about the work of John Galt and others who wanted to improve their lives. Since then the government has done more and more to try to ensure the health and welfare of its people. This has been an expensive business.

Governments now spend more on health, welfare and pensions than on education, defence and all other matters put together. It is for voters and their politicians to decide whether this spending continues to rise and to do all they can to get value for the money as they try to look after the people's health.

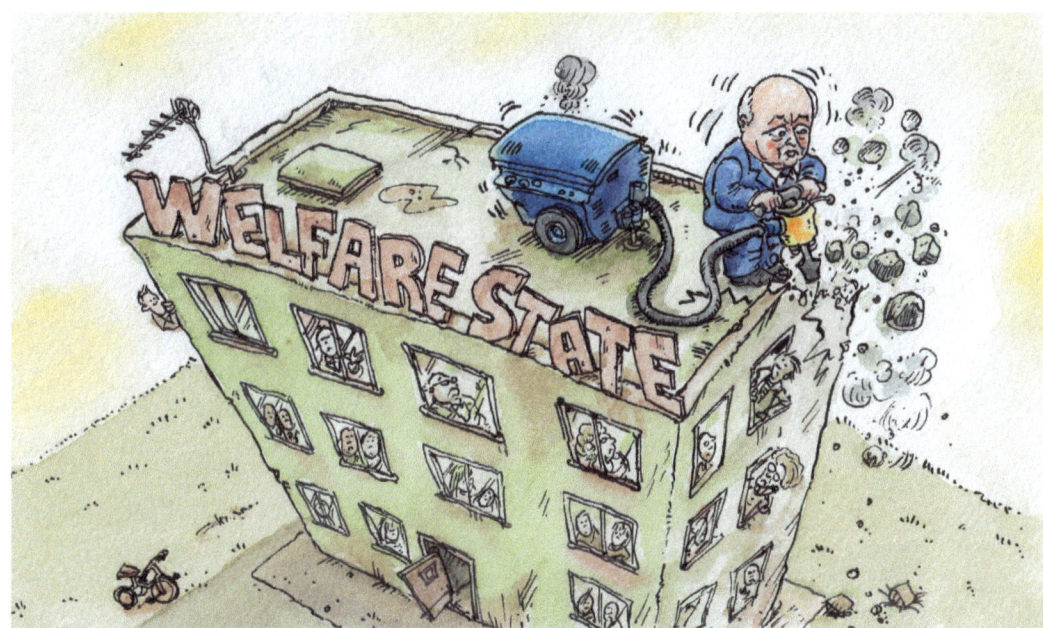

◀ This cartoon from 2013 shows a government minister dismantling a building that represents the Welfare State. Its occupants look out in dismay.

Review

You have been considering whether the story of public health in the twentieth century has been a story of progress. You have made notes about both sides of this issue. But it is never enough just to look at both sides of an argument. You have to weigh up the evidence and reach a conclusion.

For each of the following issues, use your notes to decide whether you think there has been progress and whether this can fairly be described as 'a simple story of progress'.

- Living conditions since 1900
- Epidemics since 1900
- Government involvement in health care since 1900

Write a clear explanation that sums up your thinking. Use examples to back up your ideas.

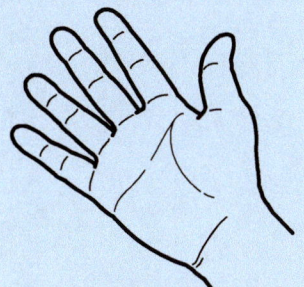

When you weigh the evidence, don't just count up which side of the argument has most notes. This is not about quantity, but quality. Which evidence is most convincing?

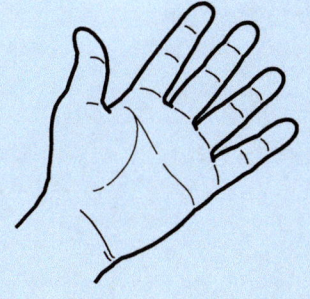

CLOSER LOOK 4

Health: a global perspective

This book is about Britain and the way it has cared for its people's health. But Britain cannot be isolated from the rest of the world. It is time to take a closer look at the global picture.

▼ Earth from space

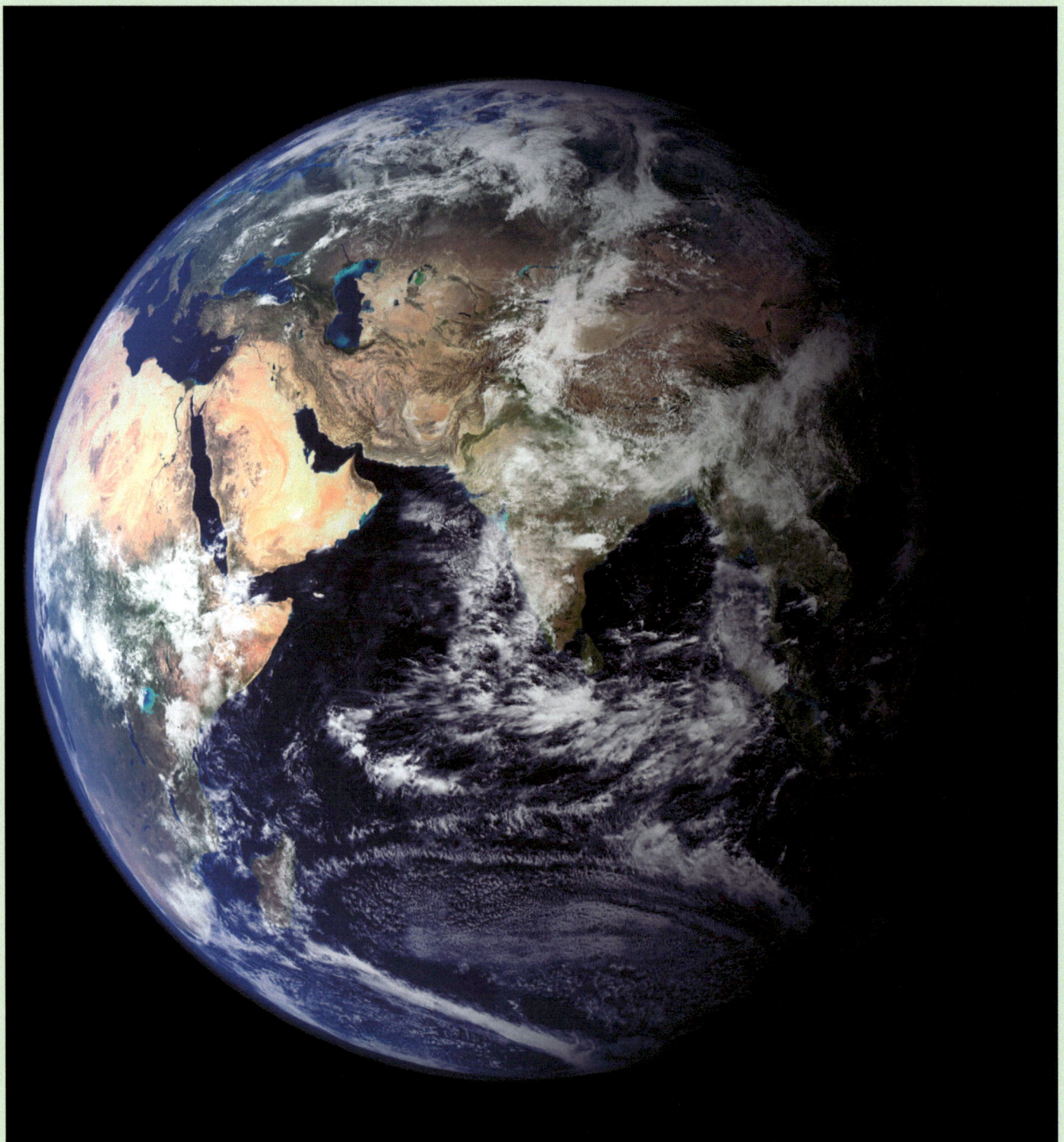

Health: a global perspective

Connections

Health issues in the wider world have always affected Britain. Think of epidemics that have arrived here from lands far away. With the arrival of modern air transport, people now move more easily than ever and so do the diseases they carry. It is almost inevitable that another virus-related disease will, at some point, spread worldwide, taking millions of lives. Britain will not be isolated from its effects.

Worldwide communications can be helpful as well, of course. Ideas on health and medicine have always moved from place to place. In the Middle Ages, the ideas of ancient Greeks were passed on to Europe from Muslim lands. In the nineteenth century, scientists in France and Germany led the way in proving that germs cause infectious diseases and in showing how vaccines can give immunity. Now, teams of medical scientists, including people of many nationalities, attend international conferences to share their findings. Britain and the rest of the world has benefited from their work.

Poverty

You will have noticed how in each period of British history it has been people who are poor who have suffered the worst conditions and had the highest rates of death. This is true on a global scale. The poorest people in the poorest countries have the lowest life expectancy. The government of each nation has the first responsibility for their care, but in 1948 the World Health Organisation (WHO) was created to help improve public health around the world. Its 2015 report included this summary:

> A staggering 1 billion people (14% of the world population) have no access to toilets, latrines or any form of sanitation facility at all and therefore practised open defecation. This leads to high levels of environmental contamination and exposure to the risks of microbial infections, diarrhoeal diseases (including cholera), trachoma, schistosomiasis and hepatitis. Around 90% of people with no access to any form of sanitation facility live in rural areas.

Alongside governments and agencies such as the WHO, churches and charities are also working hard to improve the living conditions and general health of those living in poverty. This is the same pattern that we have seen in Britain throughout this book. But there is a new threat.

The planet

In the remarkable photograph on the left, you can see a very thin light blue haze around the world. This is Earth's atmosphere. All life on the planet depends on this fragile layer of gases. Over the last century the gases have been trapping more heat and the average temperature on Earth has been rising. Unless this global warming stops, the world will change in ways that will have serious consequences for health. In different parts of the planet, water supplies will dry up, harvests will fail, air will be more polluted, insects such as ticks and mosquitoes will move into new areas, bringing disease with them. In dealing with these challenges of the future, the world may need to draw on the lessons of the past.

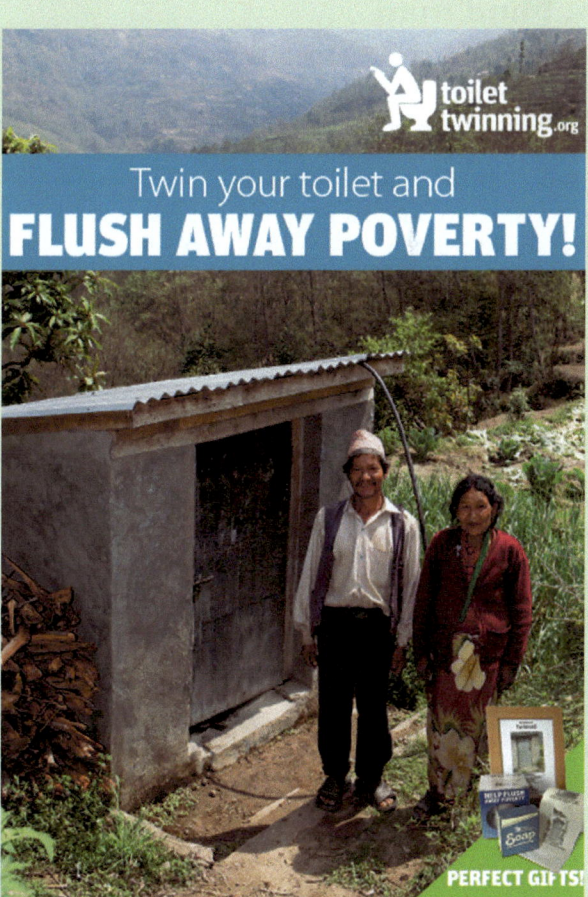

▲ A promotional leaflet for a charity that supports public health in poorer nations

Preparing for the examination

The thematic study forms the first half of Paper 1: British History. It is worth 20 per cent of your GCSE. To succeed in the examination you will need to think clearly about different aspects of the People's Health and to support your ideas with accurate knowledge. This section suggests some revision strategies and explains the types of examination questions which you can expect.

 Period summaries

Your study of the People's Health in Britain has covered four periods of history. You began each period with an overview of life in each period, then focussed on three issues:

1. Living conditions and how they affected health
2. Epidemics and how people at the time responded to them
3. How governments and others in authority attempted to improve public health

To prepare for the examination it will help to produce clear and accurate summary notes for each period. Here are four suggestions for structuring your revision notes. Choose the one which is best for you, or use a variety if you prefer.

1. Mind map

A mind map on A3 paper is a good way to summarise the important points for a particular period. A mind map will allow you to show connections between different points. It would be a good idea to use different colours for the overview and each of the three main issues.

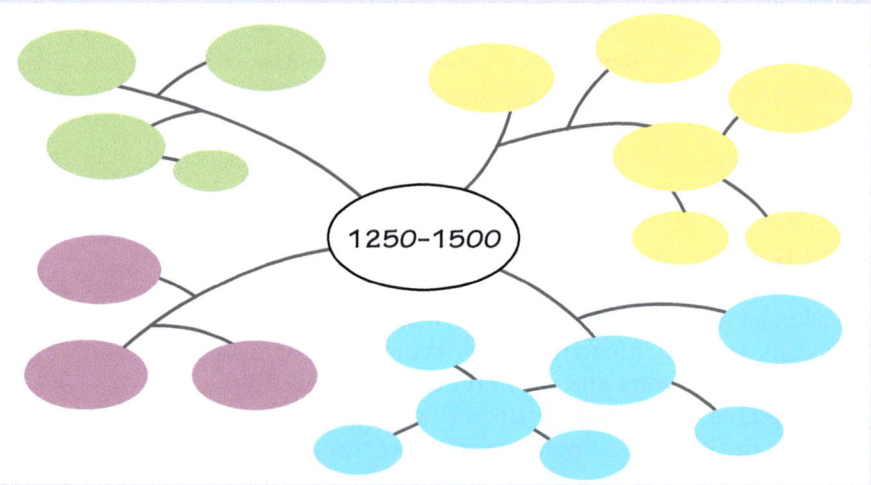

2. Chart

If you find it easier to learn information from lists, then a summary chart for each period might be best for you. You can use the format shown or design your own. Just make sure you included summary points for the overviews and each of the three main issues.

1500–1750	Overview • • •	
Living conditions • • •	Epidemics • • •	Improvements • • •

3. Small cards

Small cards are a flexible way to make revision notes. You could create sets of revision cards for the overview and for each of the three main issues. It would be a good idea to use a different colour for each set of cards.

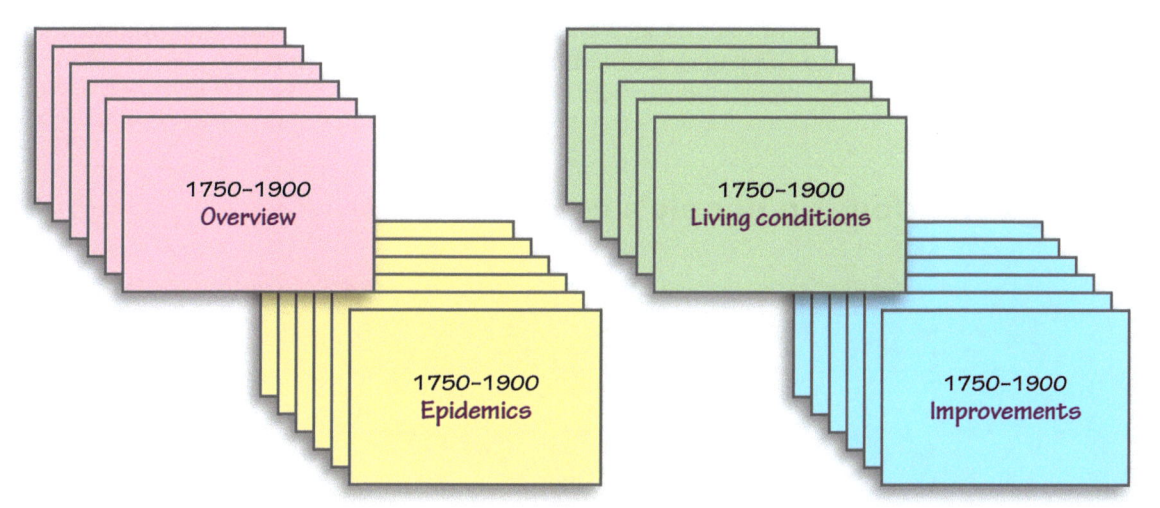

4. Podcasts

If you learn best by listening to information, you could record your knowledge and understanding of a particular period, producing podcasts to summarise the overview and each of the three issues. You could produce your podcast with a friend, using a question and answer format.

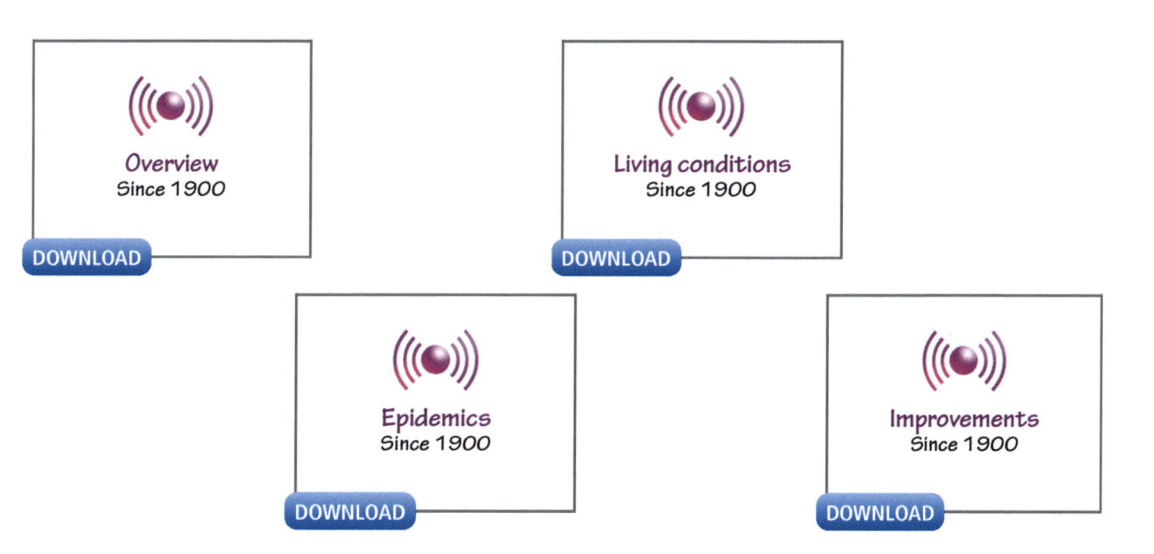

To be well-prepared for the examination you need revision notes which summarise the main points and provide detailed examples in a format that you find works best for you.

Changes and continuities

To prepare for the examination, you will need to be clear about the ways in which the people's health changed (and stayed the same) from 1250 to the present.

Some of the changes and continuities in each of three issues are shown on the timelines below. Use the notes you have made for each enquiry to produce your own detailed summary of the changes and continuities in each issue. You might find it helpful to refer to the pages detailed in the table on the right.

The impact of living conditions on people's health

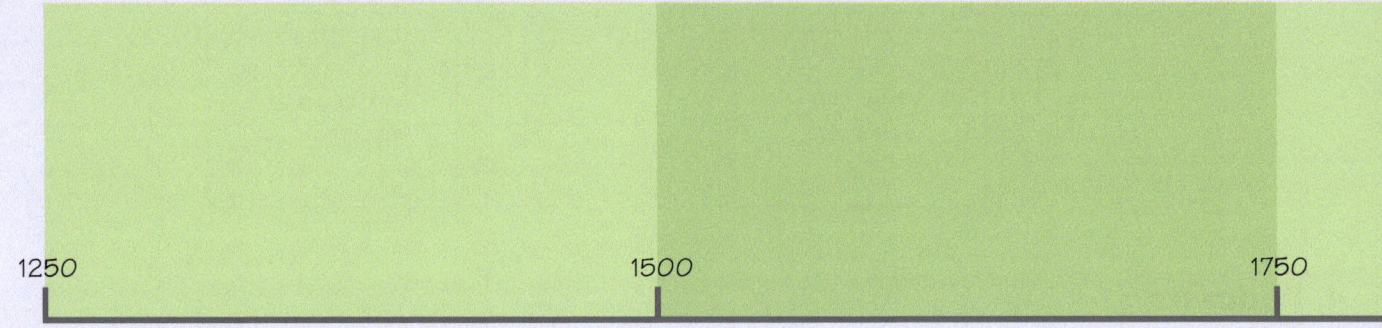

The response to epidemics

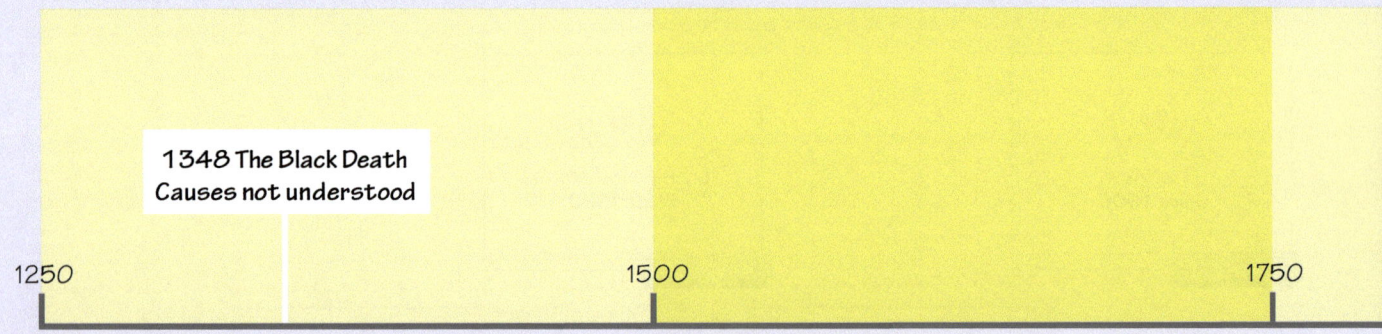

1348 The Black Death
Causes not understood

Attempts to improve public health

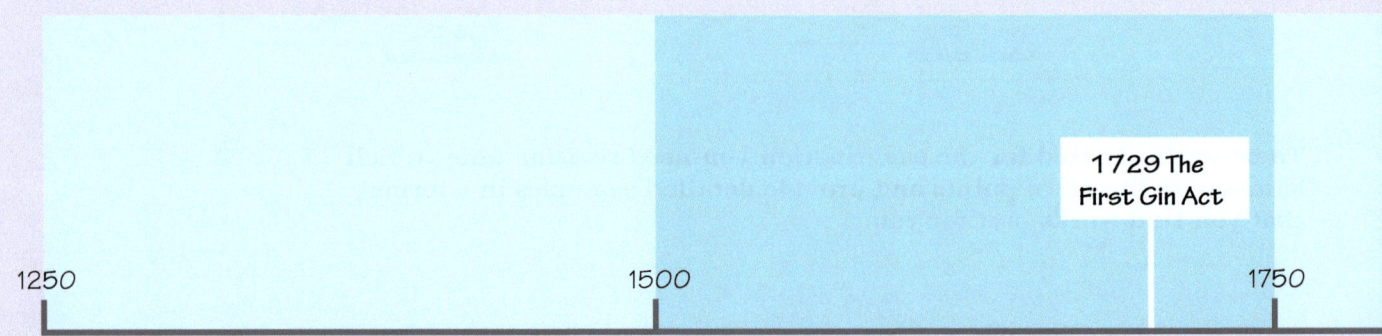

1729 The First Gin Act

Preparing for the examination

	Medieval	Early Modern	Industrial	Since 1900
Living conditions	14–19	36–41	60–63	82–87
Epidemics	20–23	42–47, 52–53	64–67	88–91
Improvements	24–29	48–51	68–75	92–95

For each issue, use your summaries to identify:
- periods of great change
- specific turning points
- periods of continuity.

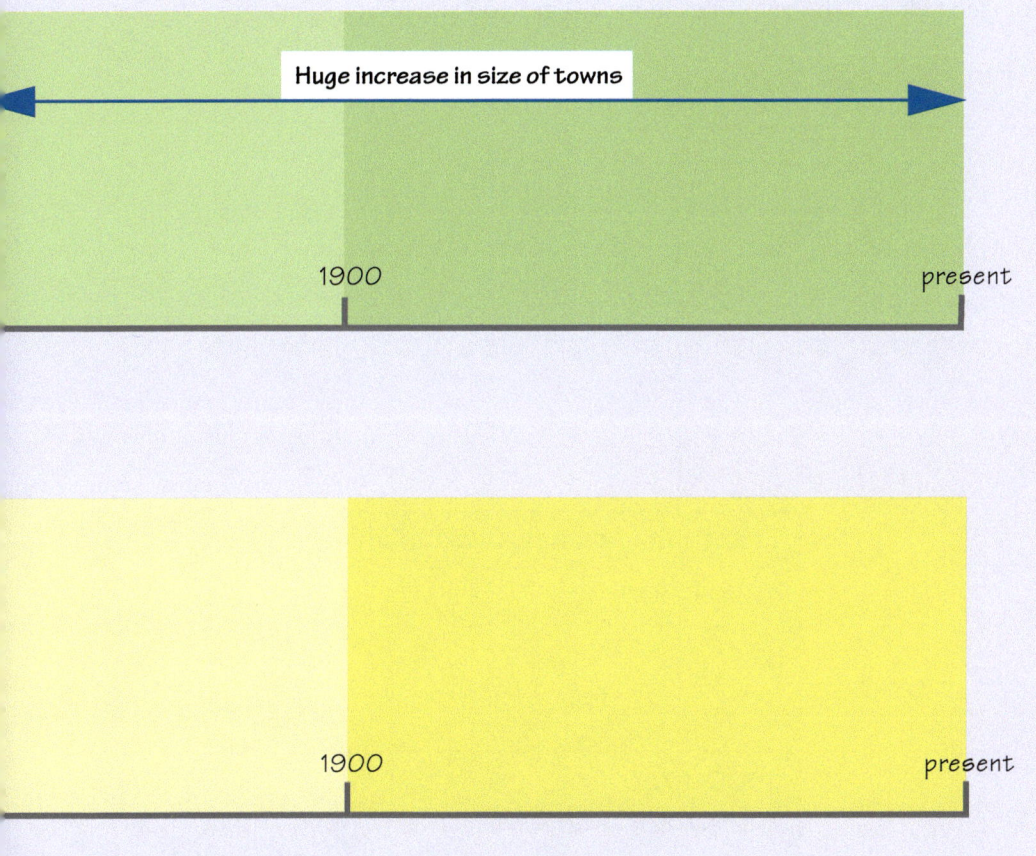

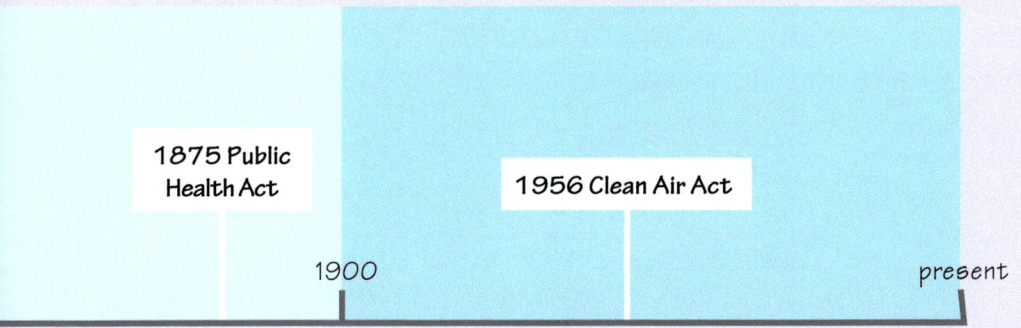

Why things changed or stayed the same

As well as explaining the patterns of change and continuity across time, historians also explain why things changed and stayed the same. Your study has focused on the ways in which the following five factors influenced changes and continuities in the people's health:

1. Beliefs, attitudes and values
2. Local and national government
3. Science and technology
4. Urbanisation
5. Wealth and poverty

Use your notes for the People's Health to create your own factor sheets with examples from different periods. It might help to use a different colour for each factor (see below). The examples here will get you started.

Beliefs, attitudes and values

1250–1500
Disease was God's punishment...

1500–1750

1750–1900

Since 1900

Local and national government

1250–1500

1500–1750
National plague orders began in 1518...

1750–1900

Since 1900

Science and technology
1250–1500
1500–1750
1750–1900 1861 – Pasteur's germ theory of disease…
Since 1900

Urbanisation
1250–1500
1500–1750
1750–1900 Rapid urbanisation – growth of major national cities…
Since 1900

Wealth and poverty
1250–1500
1500–1750
1750–1900
Since 1900 Increasing affluence after 1960…

Exam guidance

The thematic study forms the first half of Paper 1: British History. It is worth 20 per cent of your GCSE. The whole exam lasts for 1 hour 45 minutes so you will have just over fifty minutes to answer the four questions on the People's Health.

Question 1

You will be asked three quick questions each worth one mark. Question 1 requires you to show factual knowledge about the People's Health. The questions will usually begin *'Give one example of ...'*, *'Name one ...'*, *'Which ... ?'*, *'Name the ...'* or *'What was ...?'*

Example

1. a Give one example of the way in which medieval people reacted to the Black Death. (1 mark)
   b Name one way in which people in towns obtained their water in the period 1500–1750. (1 mark)
   c Name one of the 'big killer diseases' in the period 1750–1900. (1 mark)

Make a list of ten questions which you think would make a good Question 1.

Question 2

This question is worth 9 marks. It will always begin 'Write a clear and organised summary that analyses ...'. You might be asked to write a narrative account of how an aspect of the People's Health changed over time or a description of an aspect of the People's Health at a particular time.

Example

2. Write a clear and organised summary that analyses people's living conditions in the Middle Ages. Support your summary with examples. (9 marks)

Think of five more good questions for the summary task.

Preparing for the examination

Question 3
This is an explanation task worth 10 marks. Typical questions will begin with 'Why … ?', 'Why did … ?', 'What was the impact of … ?', 'What caused … ?', 'Why do you think … ?'

Example

3 Why did people's attempts to stop the spread of plague in the period 1500–1750 have limited impact? Support your answer with examples.

(10 marks)

Think of five more good questions for the explanation task.

Question 4/5
You have a choice of two judgement questions, Question 4 or Question 5. These questions in the first part of Paper 1 are the most challenging because they ask you to make a judgement about an aspect of the People's Health. You need to save enough time for the judgement question because it is worth 18 marks. The question will always ask you 'How far' you agree with a given statement.

Examples

4 How far do you agree that the most important changes in public health in Britain took place in the twentieth century? Give reasons for your answer. (18 marks)
5 'New technology has been the most important factor in improving public health in Britain.' How far do you agree with this statement? Give reasons for your answer. (18 marks)

Think of five more good questions for the judgement task.

Glossary

alderman a member of an English council elected by other members or by popular vote

allotment small plot of land often used for growing vegetables

antibiotics group of drugs used to treat infections caused by bacteria

apothecaries chemists

apprentice someone learning a craft

aqueduct channel that carries water, often over long distances and across valleys

archaeologist someone who learns about the past by finding and studying remains of objects and buildings

archives historical records and documents

bronchitis a disease that makes breathing difficult

carter a person who drives a cart

cess pit a pit or chamber used for collecting human excrement

civil registration official recording of information e.g. about dates of birth and death

colonies an area of land controlled and often inhabited by people from another country

conduit a small fountain or water pipe

coroner an official who investigates violent deaths

corporations a group of people elected to run a town or organisation

council a group of people elected to run local government

courts as in 'courtyard', a small area around which houses were built

crucified being executed by being nailed to a wooden cross

dearth lack of food e.g. after a bad harvest

delirious excited and out of control

epidemic a disease that affects a large number of people at the same time

ergotism a terrible human disease caused by fungus growing on crops

factor something that plays a part in causing an event or development

faeces excrement, solid human waste

famine desperate shortage of food

fasting choosing to go without food for a period of time

flagellants people who whip themselves or others e.g. to try to avoid getting the plague

flu see influenza

four humours four liquids that make up the human body, according to ancient Greek doctors

gluttony greed, especially for food

gongfermer person who cleans out cesspits

guilds organisations that control how a trade is run e.g. setting standards and prices

hallucination seeing things that do not really exist

hazard something that presents a risk

humanist person who believes humans are fully responsible for their own lives without God

hygiene keeping clean

immunise helping bodies resist infectious diseases

industrialisation the development of industry, involving the growth of factories and cities

inflammation swelling or soreness

Influenza a disease that involves a fever, caused by a virus

isolation being alone e.g. to avoid spreading diseases to other people

laissez-faire allowing people to look after their own affairs without government involvement

latrine toilet without any flushing system

lepers people suffering from the skin disease called leprosy

malnourished underfed or the failure to eat enough healthy foods

mayor the official in charge of a town

medieval from the Middle Ages

miasma an invisible mist that was once thought to cause diseases

microbe tiny living creature that causes disease, too small to be seen by the eye

midden a dunghill or pile of rubbish

middling sort people in the middle of society, neither rich nor poor

midwives women who assist mothers giving birth

mill a factory

obesity being extremely overweight

paviours worker who lays paving stones in streets

pesthouses buildings outside the city walls where plague victims were made to stay

pestilence any serious infectious disease

physicians trained doctors

plague a disease that first appeared in England as the Black Death in 1348

pottage a thick vegetable soup

privy toilet, often without any flushing system

psychiatrist someone who treats people's mental disorders

public health measures taken by governments and other authorities to look after people's health

quarantine being kept away from other people for a period of time to prevent the spread of a disease

rancid food that has gone bad and smells

raker street cleaner

rates taxes paid to local authorities

rickets a disease that involves the softening of the bones

sacred holy

sanitary inspector official who had to check that standards of hygiene were kept especially in shops

secular non-religious; to do with human affairs without any involvement of God or the church

sensuality enjoyment of physical pleasures e.g. food and sex

sewerage a system for draining away waste including human excrement and urine

sickle a hand-tool with a curved blade for cutting crops or hedges

slums dirty and overcrowded housing

smog dense fog mixed with fumes from cars or factories

supernatural to do with forces such as gods or spirits

tanner person who treats animal skins to make leather

terraced a row e.g. houses joined end to end

transportation system for taking prison convicts to spend years away from home in a distant land

urban to do with towns or cities

urbanisation the rapid growth of towns and cities

vendor seller

water-borne diseases diseases that are spread by microbes living in water, e.g. cholera

water closet a flushing toilet

Welfare State system by which a government takes responsibility for the health and well-being of the people

yards as in 'courtyard', a small area around which houses were built

Index

AIDS 90-1, 97
air pollution 18, 37, 54, 86
alcohol 50, 59
ale 15, 17, 35, 50
alehouses 35, 50
animals
    butchering 18, 26
    in towns 38
antibiotics 79, 85
apothecaries 47
attitudes *see* beliefs, attitudes and values

Baker, Dr Robert 66
Bath 33
Bazalgette, Joseph 70, 74-5
beer 15, 35, 50
beliefs, attitudes and values
    medieval England 10-11, 22
    1500-1750 34, 46-7
    1750-1900 67, 72
    1900-2000 78, 79
Black Death 20-3
Booth, Charles 77
bread 14, 16, 36, 37
Bristol 25, 33, 42
British Empire 57
bubonic plague 21, 43

Cambridge 43, 45
camomile 21
Carlisle 25
cars 86, 87
cesspits 16, 19, 41, 49, 66
Chadwick, Edwin 68-9
cholera 55, 64-7, 70, 71
Church
    medieval 10-11, 22, 23, 24, 28
    1500-1750 34, 46
cleanliness 40
coal 33, 56, 86
conduits 17, 41
consumption 64
cost, of a healthy society 95
countryside, life in the 11, 14-16, 32, 56
Crossness Pumping Station, London 75

Darwin, Charles 58
diarrhoea 42, 61
diet *see* food
diphtheria 42, 64
Disraeli, Benjamin 71
drink 13, 15, 41, 50-1, 59
drunkenness 13, 17, 50
dysentery 20, 42

education 58
epidemics
    AIDS 90-1
    cholera 55, 64-7, 70, 71
    plague 20-3, 30-1, 42-7, 52-3
    Spanish 'flu 88-9
ergotism 14
Exeter, medieval water supplies 28-9

famine 37
farming 11, 14, 32, 56
fish 15, 36
fleas 20, 43
food
    medieval 14-15
    1500-1750 36-7
    1750-1900 56, 61, 71
    1900-2000 84-5
Fountains Abbey, Yorkshire 24

Galt, John 77
gardens 16, 19, 24
germs 34, 58, 71
gin 50-1, 59
global health issues 96-7
gongfermers 19, 26
government
    medieval 11, 23
    1500-1750 35, 44, 50
    1750-1900 59, 67, 68-9, 70-1, 72
    1900-2000 78, 79, 82, 83, 92-5
    see also local government
Great Plague 1665 30-1, 42-3
'Great Stink' 1858 70

historical context 9
HIV 90
Hooke, Robert 34
houses and housing
    medieval 16, 19
    1500-1750 39
    1750-1900 60-1, 73
    1900-2000 82-3
human rights 79
human waste 17, 19, 41, 63, 71

inactivity 87
industrialisation 56-7
industry 18, 32-3
inequality 59
influenza 42, 64, 88-9

jakes 41, 63, 71

kings 11, 35

labourers 11, 14, 36-7
landowners 11, 34, 35, 82
latrines 17, 19, 26, 97
Leeds 60-1, 65-6
leisure 13, 80, 81
life expectancy 42, 64
living conditions
    medieval 14-19
    1500-1750 36-41
    1750-1900 57, 60-3
    1900-2000 82-7
local government
    medieval 13, 25-6, 29
    1500-1750 45, 48-9
    1750-1900 59, 60, 67, 72-3
    1900-2000 82, 83
London
    medieval 26
    1500-1750 30-1, 49
    1750-1900 57, 69, 74-5
lords, medieval 11
Luttrell Psalter 9

Manchester 54, 72-3
markets 17
measles 42, 64
miasma 22, 43, 63, 67
middens 16, 63, 71
monasteries 10, 24, 34

national government *see* government
National Health Service (NHS) 92, 93
Newcastle 52-3
Newcomen, Thomas 33
newspapers 58
night soil men 63
Niven, Dr James 89
Norwich 25

Pacini, Filippo 70
pail privies 71
Palfreyman, James 54-5
parliament 35, 59
Pasteur, Louis 58, 60, 71
peasants 11, 14, 16
physicians 47
plague 20-3, 30-1, 42-7, 52-3
Plague Act 1604 44
plague orders 44, 48
pneumonia 42
pneumonic plague 21
pollution 18, 37, 86
population 56, 80, 81
pottage 16, 37
poverty
    medieval 11, 16, 19

1550–1750 35, 36–7, 50
1750–1900 59, 60–1, 68
1900–2000 77, 80, 87
printing press 34, 44
privies 41, 63, 71
public health, defined 8
Public Health Act 1848 69
Public Health Act 1875 71
Pure Food Act 1860 71

railways 57
rakers 17, 19, 41
rats 20, 43
Reform Act 1832 59
Reform Act 1867 71
religion
    medieval 10, 22
    1500–1750 46
    1750–1900 58
    1900–2000 78, 79
rickets 85
roads and streets 17, 37
Rowntree, Seebohm 77

scarlet fever 42
scavengers 41
science
    medieval 12
    1500–1750 34
    1750–1900 58, 70
    1900–2000 78, 79, 84
septicemic plague 21

sewage 63, 70
sewers 63, 69, 74–5
Shrewsbury 25
Simon, John 70
smallpox 42
smells 18, 70
smog 86
smoke 39, 86
smoking, tobacco 93–4
Snow, John 70
Spanish 'flu 88–9
steam engines 33
streets and roads 17, 38
syphilis 42

Tailor, Ralph 52, 53
technology
    medieval 12
    1500–1750 33, 34
    1750–1900 57
    1900–2000 78, 79, 81, 84, 87
textile industry 12, 15, 32, 56, 57
toilets 41, 63, 69, 97
towns
    medieval 13, 17–19, 23, 25–6, 29
    1500–1750 33, 35, 38–9, 44, 45, 48–9
    1750–1900 54–5, 57, 60–3, 67
trade 12, 33, 57
tuberculosis 64
typhoid 42, 60, 64, 75
typhus 42, 64

urban environment *see* towns
values *see* beliefs, attitudes and values
van Leeuwenhoek, Antonie 34
villages 13, 15–16

waste
    medieval 16, 17, 19
    1500–1750 41
    1750–1900 63, 70, 71, 74–5
water closets 41, 63, 69
water mills 12, 15
water and water supplies
    medieval 15, 17, 19, 24, 28–9
    1500–1750 40–1
    1750–1900 62, 72–3
wealth
    medieval 11, 16, 19
    1500–1750 35, 36, 40–1
    1750–1900 59
    1900–2000 80, 81, 87
Welfare State 78, 79, 93
Winchester 25
windmills 12
witchcraft 34
Women's Co-operative Guild 72
wool 12, 32
work and workers 11, 32, 56, 80, 81
World Health Organisation (WHO) 97
Wrightson, Keith 52, 53

Yersima pestis 20
York 25, 44, 48, 77

Acknowledgements

Text acknowledgements: p.97 Reprinted from 'World Health Statistics 2015, Goal 7, Target 7.C: Halve, by 2015, the proportion of the population without sustainable access to safe drinking water and basic sanitation', page 23, Copyright (2015).

Photo credits: pp.6-7 © Alex Segre / Alamy Stock Photo; **p.8** The Black Death (gouache on paper), Nicolle, Pat (Patrick) (1907-95)/Private Collection/© Look and Learn/Bridgeman Images/Bridgeman Images; **p.9** © British Library/The Art Archive; **p.10** *t* © The British Library Board (Add. 42130, f.44); **p.10** *b* Psalm 37; nun's confession/British Library, London, UK/© British Library Board. All Rights Reserved/Bridgeman Images; **p.11** *t* © The British Library Board (Add. 42130, f.16v); **p.11** *m* © PBL Collection/Alamy Stock Photo; **p.11** *b* © British Library/The Art Archive; **p.12** *t* © The British Library Board (Add. 42130, f.158); **p.12** *m* © British Library/akg-images; **p.12** *b* © British Library/akg-images; **p.13** *t* © British Library/akg-images; **p.13** *b* Psalm 83; fighting with pitchers/© British Library Board. All Rights Reserved/Bridgeman Images; **p.14** *t* 42130 f.172v Peasants harvesting, begun prior to 1340 for Sir Geoffrey Luttrell (1276-1345), Latin (vellum), English School, (14th century)/British Library, London, UK/© British Library Board. All Rights Reserved/Bridgeman Images; **p.14** *b* © Gianni Dagli Orti/Unterlinden Museum Colmar/The Art Archive; **p.15** © British Library/akg-images; **p.16** *t* © Historic England/Mary Evans; **p.17** *t* © The Art Archive/Alamy Stock Photo; **p.17** *b* © British Library/The Art Archive; **p.18** *t* © The British Library Board (Add. 42130, f.159v); **p.19** *t* © Homer Sykes/Alamy Stock Photo; **p.19** *b* © Odense City Museums; **p.20** *b* Ms 89 fol.88 The Triumph of Death, from a Book of Hours (vellum), French School, (15th century)/© Bibliotheque Municipale, Moulins, France/Bridgeman Images; **p.22** © World History Archive/Alamy Stock Photo; **p.23** © V&A Images/Alamy Stock Photo; **p.24** © The Historic England Archive, Historic England; **p.25** Medieval Deeds (ink on paper), English School/© Chetham's Library, Manchester, UK/Bridgeman Images; **p.27** © Mary Evans Picture Library; **p.28** *t* © Exeter Underground Passages; **p.28** *b* Courtesy Dean & Chapter of Exeter Cathedral; **p.29** © Exeter Archaeology, Drawn by P. Bishop; **p.30-1** Wikimedia; **p.32** *t* Country Round Dixton Manor, c.1725 (oil on canvas) (detail of 18102), English School, (18th century)/© Cheltenham Art Gallery & Museums, Gloucestershire, UK/Bridgeman Images; **p.32** *b* © The Granger Collection, NYC/TopFoto; **p.33** *t* © Classic Image/Alamy; **p.33** *m* © The Granger Collection, NYC/TopFoto; **p.33** *b* © Bath in Time – Bath Preservation Trust Collection; **p.34** *t* © Robert Harding Picture Library Ltd/Alamy; **p.34** *m* © Wellcome Library, London. Wellcome Images; **p.34** *b* Hanging of witches/British Library, London, UK/© British Library Board. All Rights Reserved/Bridgeman Images; **p.35** *t* © World History Archive/Alamy; **p.35** *m* The Tichborne Dole, 1671, Tilborgh, Gillis van (1625-78)/© Tichborne House, Hampshire, UK/Bridgeman Images; **p.35** *b* © Chronicle/Alamy; **p.36** © Eileen Tweedy/Marquess of Bath/The Art Archive; **p.38-9** © Ivan Lapper; **p.40** *t* © London Metropolitan Archives, City of London; **p.40** *b* © Guildhall Library & Art Gallery/Heritage Images/Getty Images; **p.41** © The Clothworker's Company; **p.42** ©Wellcome Library, London/http://creativecommons.org/licenses/by/4.0/; **p.43** ©Wellcome Library, London/http://creativecommons.org/licenses/by/4.0/; **p.45** *t* © The Granger Collection, NYC/TopFoto; **p.45** *b* Reproduced by the kind permission of the Syndics of Cambridge University Library; **p.46** © Timewatch Images/Alamy; **p.47** ©Wellcome Library, London/http://creativecommons.org/licenses/by/4.0/; **p.48** © Hulton Archive/Getty Images; **p.49** *t* © London Metropolitan Archives, City of London; **p.49** *b* © Heritage Image Partnership Ltd /Alamy; **p.50** ©The Bodleian Library, University of Oxford (shelfmark: Douce HH.227); **p.51** ©Wellcome Library, London/http://creativecommons.org/licenses/by/4.0/; **p.52** *t* Reproduced courtesy of Yale University Press London; **p.53** *r* © Newcastle City Library; **p.53** *l* Reproduced by permission of Durham University Library; **p.54-5** © Mary Evans Picture Library/Alamy Stock Photo; **p.56** *t* ©Universal History Archive/UIG/Getty Images; **p.56** *b* ©Mary Evans Picture Library; **p.57** *t* ©SSPL/Getty Images; **p.57** *m* Imperial Federation (colour litho), Crane, Walter (1845-1915) (after)/Private Collection/© Look and Learn/Bridgeman Images; **p.57** *b* © Mary Evans Picture Library; **p.58** *t* © Illustrated London News Ltd/Mary Evans; **p.58** *m* © The Granger Collection, New York/TopFoto; **p.58** *b* Advertisements (engraving), English School, (19th century)/Private Collection/© Look and Learn/Illustrated Papers Collection/Bridgeman Images; **p.59** *t* © TP Archive/ILN/Mary Evans Picture Library; **p.59** *m* Poverty and Wealth, 1888 (oil on canvas), Frith, William Powell (1819-1909)/Private Collection/Photo © Peter Nahum at The Leicester Galleries, London/Bridgeman Images; **p.59** *b* © Mary Evans Picture Library; **p.61** Courtesy of Manchester Libraries, Information and Archives, Manchester City Council; **p.62** © Wellcome Library, London. Wellcome Images/http://creativecommons.org/licenses/by/4.0/; **p.63** © Mary Evans Picture Library; **p.65** © Leeds Library and Information Service, Leodis; **p.66** © Thackray Medical Museum; **p.68** © London Stereoscopic Company/Getty Images; **p.69** © Wellcome Library, London. Wellcome Images/http://creativecommons.org/licenses/by/4.0/; **p.70** © TopFoto; **p.71** © Unknown photographer/Science & Society Picture Library; **p.72** © By permission of The People's History Museum, Manchester; **p.73** *t* © TopFoto.co.uk; **p.73** *b* © Mike Robinson/Alamy Stock Photo; **p.74** *t* © Print Collector/HIP/TopFoto; **p.75** *t* © W. Brown/Otto Herschan/Getty Images; **p.75** *b* © Eric Nathan/Alamy Stock Photo; **p.76** © Museum of London/Heritage Images/Getty Images); **p.77** © Heritage Image Partnership Ltd/Alamy Stock Photo; **p.78** *t* © University of Bristol Library, Special Collections; **p.78** *m* © Time Life Pictures/Mansell/The LIFE Picture Collection/Getty Images; **p.78** *b* © Past Pix/SSPL/Science and Society/Superstock; **p.79** *t* © Justin Kase z09z/Alamy Stock Photo; **p.79** *m* © dpa picture alliance/Alamy Stock Photo; **p.79** *b* ©Peter Bates/Getty Images; **p.80** *t* © AS400 DB/Corbis; **p.80** *m* ©TopFoto; **p.80** *b* © Chronicle/Alamy Stock Photo; **p.81** *t* Mark Bowden/Thinkstock/iStock/Getty Images; **p.81** *m* © Gideon Mendel/Corbis; **p.81** *b* © Radharc Images/Alamy Stock Photo; **p.83** *t* © Bristol Record Office: BRO 40826/HSG/52; **p.83** *m* © The Russell Butcher Collection/Mary Evans Picture Library; **p.84** Reproduced by permission of Surrey Libraries (Ewell); **p.85** ©SSPL/Getty Images; **p.86** © Monty Fresco/Getty Images; **p.87** *t* © Jonty Clark; **p.87** *b* © Jeff Morgan 08/Alamy Stock Photo; **p.88** © Topical Press Agency/Getty Images; **p.89** © Hardy Pictures; **p.90** © Stocktrek Images/Superstock; **p.91** ©Anwar hussein/Getty Images; **p.93** © 20th Century Advertising/Alamy Stock Photo; **p.95** © Dave Simonds; **p.96** © NASA Goddard NASA/Space Flight Center Image by Reto Stöckli (land surface, shallow water, clouds). Enhancements by Robert Simmon (ocean color, compositing, 3D globes, animation). Data and technical support: MODIS Land Group; MODIS Science Data Support Team; MODIS Atmosphere Group; MODIS Ocean Group Additional data: USGS EROS Data Center (topography); USGS Terrestrial Remote Sensing Flagstaff Field Center (Antarctica); Defense Meteorological Satellite Program (city lights); **p.97** © Toilet Twinning (www.toilettwinning.org).